Miracles of Nutrition

Miracles of Nutrition

Descending Eagle

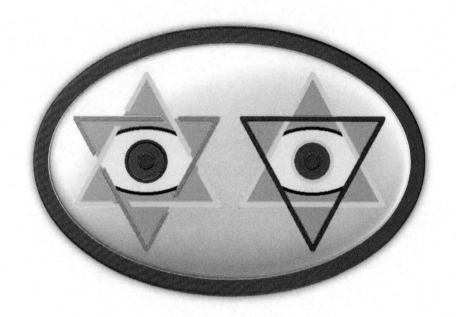

8th Book of Life

Nebulous Henctis

Publisher: Living Tree Services
Published in 2005
ISBN# 978-1-965502-03-7

To the Angel of the Church of Laodicea

Ashes and Manna in Marble and Silver

Thank GOD for revealing the keys and sharing how to bring them together.

Thanks to family, friends, and everyone else who helped gather and assemble the keys.

And to the Soul Coach who helped gather the information in this book, thank you, Ora.

Table of Contents

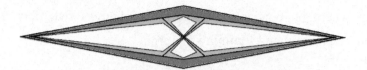

Introduction
Quantum Healing

Throughout this world, there are many types of coaches. There are sports coaches, career coaches, financial coaches, and many other types. This book is for spiritual coaching of the Way. The goal is to heal, transform, and empower your entire being.

Here you will find a resourceful and modern map of the frequencies of the new Earth. Step by step, this book is like an atlas for fine-tuning each area within your life. Descending Eagle has many types of nourishing information, including studies on energetics, food, bodybuilding, and more. It is intended to help your personal spiritual growth.

Book 8, Miracles of Nutrition, is designed in conjunction with Oracles of Time Book 7 in this series. Together they can help you activate and divinely align your entire life path.

Book 7 of this series presents that Jesus is now in charge in heaven and that heaven includes the Zodiac systems with guidance for all religions. The astrological calendars are a combined celestial map of the terrestrial heavens. (Matthew 28:18) (Philippians 3:20)

Now, in Book 8, the focus turns to the energies of your personal auric field. You are provided with an in-depth educational experience on how to cleanse your energies and become the best version of yourself. These energies were mentioned in Book 7.

Here is an excerpt from Book 7 of this series, Oracles of Time, Ascending Ram.

When someone is connected to a polygraph machine, their blood pressure, pulse, respiration, and skin conductivity are measured. These measurements resemble a wave on a graph. Similarly, we measure vibrations with seismographs and helicorders. We can even monitor our emotions and thoughts.

Each person has unique biophysical oscillations and vibrations, which can change due to interactions with their surroundings. These are our physical frequencies.

Personality offset begins when the conception of a fetus receives two sets of chromosomes: genetic contributions from masculine paternal and feminine maternal.

When paternal and maternal genetic imprints merge, their bio-physical oscillations unite. Fusing impressions conceive one bio-physical fingerprint with its own oscillations.

The parents interact from moment to moment throughout pregnancy. Dad continues to cause fluctuations in Mom while fetal development continues.

Interactions from outside the parents fluctuate upon their energies, entering within the growing embryo, which absorbs surrounding vibrations. Mom contacts her surroundings and other people. Dad also does. The parents intermingle with people who have their own biophysical oscillations. Populations are networks of these fluctuating energies. Social connections adjust Mom and Dad as they experience and learn within their surrounding environments.

When the Dad eases and calms the Mom's emotions, her moods cause bio-fluctuations through the fetus' maturation. Even micro energetic and magnetic energies and stimulants, regardless of how minute they may seem, continue to embrace the nature of the nurtured fetus.

End of excerpt.

These energy fields that surround us are what some people call auras. Some say that they can see them. The scientific simplicity behind seeing auras is in comprehending synesthesia. This possibly rare ability called synesthesia happens when one sensory system in the body crosses over to another sensory system. The nervous and synapse systems in the minds of people with synesthesia can be connected differently. They have links that allow diverse abilities. They may see sounds or taste colors. People also have spiritual senses and can sense Spirit. If your perception of the Spirit synesthetically crosses over your perception of vision, you may see auras.

When someone enters a church or any other type of spiritual group, they often feel a comforting energy. This energy can be referred to as a good vibe. This vibe comes from the energy fields of the groups of people gathered together. Most people can feel the vibe of a group or even a single person. Those who can see auras have a form of synesthesia that allows them to see the vibrational frequency radiating from within the person. Auras have often been seen in color form.

For those who cannot visually see auras, there is another way to view them. Each of these energy vibrations is categorized in an organizational system called chakras. The chakra system was designed to educate us in the process of increasing and/or evolving our vibrations. Each chakra vibration is associated with a color.

The chakras in this book are correctly aligned with the Urim and Thummim. The Urim and Thummim is explained in detail within Book 7 of this series.

The purpose of this information is to help you elevate your spiritual practices. Though this book discusses many religious ideas, these coaching practices are not a religion. You may know GOD as Source, Creator, or by another understanding. Of these mentioned, GOD is the most common view expressed in this book.

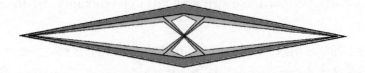

Chapter 1
Learning your Frequency – Starseed of Abraham

This first chapter explains terminology and ideas commonly used when discussing subjects of the spiritual quantum field. The information relates to cleansing energies for becoming lightworkers and starseeds. All of it can be used for the betterment of your soul.

Quantum Field – This term means the realm of physics in which the known universe operates within. It is also a spiritual realm. You, as a spirit being, came to physical existence and have entered a body. Your experience is given place within the quantum field where Spirit and physical matter interact. Physics can be used to reflect upon scientific proof with explanations that include spirituality.

This is a realm of vibrational frequency. It exists within and throughout all things and is connected to your aura. Your aura interrelates through quantum substances that are material and spiritual. Physical and spiritual vibrations are both factors in our evolutionary experience.

Quantum frequencies can be felt if you are tuned into sensing them. They are different from emotions, yet they are aspects of how your emotions fluctuate and vice versa. They help shape your emotions and emotions help shape them.

In the Quantum Field, you can diagnose and make changes within the physical/spiritual mainframe of the people. Here you can touch and handle both physical and spiritual matter. You can enter humanity here and help reconnect their spirit(s) to GOD.

Energetics – This form of the word energetics means the scientific and spiritual abilities of energies, including the ways that they are merged and distributed through humanity and the cosmos.

Your energetics are your ability to make shifts within reality using your spiritual and physical energies. Your physical existence is a formula of energetic substance. Your thoughts are energy. Your emotions are energy. Your actions are energetic expressions. You can distribute the essence of your energy into the collective consciousness of humanity and into the entire universe. This is done with energetic chemistry. Everything you do redirects into your surroundings. Your thoughts, emotions, and actions blend with the united energy of the cosmos. Your ways make a difference throughout all existence.

Energy – This form of the word energy means the property that is manifest as the capacity to propel thoughts, feelings, and actions. Energy comes in many forms. You have spiritual energy and physical energy. Your main forms of energy are emotional energy, physical energy, doctrinal energy, spiritual energy, mental energy, soul energy, social energy, and the energy of your works. Together they are your energetic way.

Vitality – This form of the word vitality means the state of your energy being strong and lively. It is your power of continuance and steadiness.

Vital Energy or Vital Life Force – These terms mean the energy source of your aura, like a battery full of life energy. Some people call this your spirit when they say things like, "she has a lot of spirit in her."

As an internal charge, your auric energy can be used to do various things. You can share your life force with anyone that you choose. Those with a lot of vital energy may have the ability to happily help many people. (Mark 5:30) (Luke 6:19, 24:49)

Your energy can also get tired, and you may need recharging. The best ways to recharge are in feeling and expressing love in peacefulness. Some people may need time alone to recharge. Being in nature is a wonderful way to refresh your vital life.

Your internal charge is based on your experiences and intellect. Unwanted experiences may have caused your internal energy to radiate undesirable feelings or pessimistic thoughts. The internal charge that you build gets stored inside your cells and DNA. Your mood affects your health.

A healthier mood translates into a healthier body. For the benefit of your own well-being, you can explore valuable charging experiences. Consider that the world is beautiful and abundant everywhere. Even those incidents that are not so pleasant are there so that you can learn. Your ability to learn is enjoyable, and therefore all things can be pleasing.

Live life as if everything is prepared in your favor. Become a magnet for all that is good in the universe. Cultivate that energy within you. Use your vital life intentionally to create what you want to experience.

You can develop divine energy. The more you elevate your energy within the Spirit, the less that an undesirable experience can adversely affect your internal charge. When you have cultivated and anchored a godly frequency, you can hold onto it even when the external world is showing you otherwise. When you can hold an elevated energy, that's when things can really open up for you. Solidify your trust in GOD.

Vibration – This form of the word vibration means a person's emotional condition or the ambiance of a place or an object, as others feel it. The voice of the frequency of the collective consciousness within the atmosphere where you reside has a vibration. This includes physical and social environments. Your vibration is the voice of your personal frequency. Your vibration allows people to feel your frequency when in your presence. Your vibration resonates your state of consciousness within your own personal atmosphere of who you are. This includes your mental, emotional, and physical states. Here you will find guidance that can help you raise your vibration to a more desirable and healthier state of consciousness. Advancing your vibration affects your DNA, atomic, and molecular structures in beneficial ways.

Frequency – This form of the word frequency means the level of the vibration of a person, place, or thing. You may have a higher or a lower vibration. Your frequency is your energetic signature. Picture your vibration as the key note of the essence of your tune and your frequency as the octave of your key note.

There are different types of frequencies. This can be noted in the difference between adrenaline and spiritual motivation. We use spiritual frequencies to speak in energetic ways. People can hear each other even in silence. That is because of the fifth-dimensional connection that people have. The energy of your aura is spiritually translated and merged into the physical.

Raw physical frequency can be in one place, vibrating an effect upon its surroundings. Spiritual frequency can be everywhere at once. The spirit can transfer information so much faster than light that it is instant from any distance. Spirit goes beyond physical and into all realms. Spiritual and physical need each other.

Activator – This form of the word activator means a person that stimulates a process of operative chemistry. An activator is someone who consciously decides to cause a happening. You can cause your energetic substance to deliberately stimulate and create a better chemistry within the conscious collective of humanity. In order to do this for others, you must first activate righteous happenings within yourself.

There are many beneficial traits to being an activator. Once they can successfully activate themselves, the energy and frequency of an activator can do things to/for those around them. Activators inspire and share beneficial things with people. They apply helpful ideas to life. They focus on beneficial progressiveness. They are producers of valuable things such as helpful ideas, thoughts, and emotions instead of living only to be a consumer. They calibrate to a healthy frequency. They make changes for the better. They can feel knowledgeable and validated in what they are while keeping an openness for the continuation of growth. Activators are a gift here. They hold a high vibrational frequency, which also raises the frequency of the earth.

Introspection – This form of the word introspection means observing and examining the mechanics of your own mental, emotional, physical, and social processes. This is the first step to becoming a starseed. Establish a knowing of your own habits and behaviors. Your introspection is very connected to doing your inner works. (James 2:17) Much more information on this is in Book 10 of this series.

Timeline – This form of the word timeline means the occurring experience that you are living. You travel through your experience as if on a road or set of tracks. You can shift onto a safer and happier path if that is your choice. The word timeline is often used in another dimensional way, which won't be discussed here.

Consider you were driving along a highway, and ahead there was soon to be an unpredictable earthquake. You were about to pass a mountainside when you began thinking about how lovely nature can be. You got out of your car and took that moment to appreciate the beauties that GOD has created. You said a prayer and then got back into your vehicle. While you were praying, an earthquake sank the road that you would have been on if you had continued without stopping to view the scenery. Because you stopped, the danger was no longer on your timeline.

We can shift timelines by cultivating a connection with GOD. (Isaiah 35:8) Your greatest timeline is your best path for your best experience. Each moment, you are heading towards your future. Realign your life story to the best path possible. Your best experience includes being your most productive, most loving, most fun, and anything else that is the greatest timeline for you and for everyone. If you choose to elevate your timeline, you may begin seeing life from above your previous ways.

Manifest your life experience into your true essence. Cultivate a real connection with yourself and with others. When your path is aligned with doing what is best for everyone, then you are on a divine timeline. Be intentional about what you are choosing to experience. GOD gave you free will to decide, and therefore your power to make a change is within you. You are also an instrument in the hands of GOD. Put your life in alignment with what you want GOD to create, and you become righteous creation in motion. Claim and choose your destiny. Make higher caliber choices.

When you approach your highest timeline, you begin to ascend. When your timeline is higher than someone else's, you have the ability to lift others. (Psalm 61:1-2) You are reality.

Recalibration – This form of the word recalibration means to realign your timeline, vibration, frequency, belief system, etc. After doing introspection, you can adjust and tune yourself. You can realign yourself to be better for someone else, such as your partner. You can realign for GOD. You can realign for the job you choose. You can also recalibrate just to become a better version of yourself.

Reflect upon what you want the world to be like. Would you like people to be honest and kind? Would you like there to be more technological and spiritual advancements? For these things to happen, you must be the change that you want to see in this world. Realize that you are the kind of person that the world wants. You are the one that everyone was waiting for.

What are you expressing to yourself and into the universe? If you want the world to change, you must be more of what you desire. Your thoughts and actions create your reality.

Learn to cultivate a connection with yourself. Write down your intentions for the future of humanity. Clearly define what you value. Develop better connections and ties to your values and desires.

Your internal pillar is the 'who you are' without anyone else telling you who to be. Cultivate the internal pillar of what you really are based on your values and desires. Do you want the world to be confident and bold? Be confident and bold. Be the authentic you that the world wants to merge with. Radiate the energy of your internal pillar. You are a gift here.

Begin expressing yourself in the frequency of the very being that you wish to be. Imagine the collective consciousness of humanity as a pool of water. Your vibration is like a droplet that creates a ripple effect through society. Be the most authentic and true form of you possible. Become resilient in continuing to move forward in the direction that you want the world to go.

Transmute and Transformation – These forms of the words transmute and transformation mean to change, convert, replace, or exchange the form, nature, or substance of anything. Once you recalibrate your life, your energy, ideas, thoughts, and actions will transmute. The purpose of the people, places, and things in your life will change. Here is an example. You may have had a spare room in your house that was being used for storage. When you recalibrate your purpose in life, your spare room may transmute into a shelter for someone in need. The very nature of your existence can change. (Job 14:14)

Transition – This form of the word transition means the process or period during the transformation or transmutation from one state or condition to another. This includes mental, emotional, physical, and any other change that may happen.

Solidify – This form of the word solidify means to strengthen or reinforce. When concrete solidifies, it gets hard and solid. Similarly, your recalibrated and transformed belief systems and frequencies must solidify after transition. It can require time for this to happen. Be patient and think your ways through. Solidify the real you, and convey your energetic expression confidently.

Anchored – This form of the word anchored means to provide a firm and immovable foundation. It includes anchoring your energy, vibration, frequency, decisions, ideas, purposes, etc. Anchor your purpose into a true position. Be immovably righteous with your good deeds and decisions.

Extrospection – This form of the word extrospection means to observe and examine the mechanics of the mental, emotional, physical, and social processes around you. Establish a knowing of the habits and behaviors of the universe and others. Your extrospection is very connected to doing your outer works. (Acts 9:36) To be able to plant your starseed, you must first use extrospection in deciding where and how to plant it.

Reciprocate – This form of the word reciprocate means to correspond, relate, communicate, and reflect with your surroundings. Reciprocation can happen in any energy form, including with people, places, and things. Giving and receiving an equilibrium of kindness is good reciprocation. After extrospection, you must reciprocate with your surroundings to be able to plant your starseed.

Validate – This form of the word validate means to affirm and recognize the value of the good attributes in a person, place, or thing. When reciprocating, it is important to recognize when you find someone or something beneficial. Good qualities should be validated. You can seek out the blessings and talents in everyone and encourage them to strengthen those areas. It is essential to know that quality validation begins within your own mind and heart.

Infusion – This form of the word infusion means to introduce and combine a validated component or quality into a person, place, or thing. When a useful quality that you need is found in someone, you should combine that quality with yours in one way or another. You can infuse other people's righteous ideas into your own. You can introduce a smile to someone, and that smile can infuse them with happiness. A happy thought can be infused into your mood just to brighten your day.

Implement – This form of the word implement means to put something into effect. It can be a thought, plan, or agreement. When you infuse a righteous aspect into your own path, you can then implement a plan to use that new aspect for the greater good. Use the quality components that you have infused into your life to implement your plans to do good deeds.

Integrate – This form of the word integrate means to bring two or more people, places, or things together into one. You can integrate advanced ideas into your current belief system(s). You can integrate what others present into what you offer. For instance, all religions can be integrated into one in Omnism.

Once you have observed yourself and your atmosphere, realize that you and your surroundings are one. Establish yourself in a new vibration. Recalibrate your energy to manifest the greater good of all. Integrate yourself with your surroundings. Imagine the world collective and its current energy. Each person that increases their own energy raises the collective frequency. Know that the more righteous you are, the more righteous your surrounding environment will become. The kinder you are, the kinder people will become. The more you take care of the earth, the more the earth can take care of you. When you extend the compassion that you have for yourself to those around you, the entire collective will be more compassionate.

Celebration – This form of the word celebration means acknowledgment, observance, or commemoration. Holy integrations are worth celebrating. Acknowledge the magnificence of your life and the lives of others. Hold observance of the wonderful gifts of GOD. Commemorate how far everyone has come together.

Transcendence – This form of the word transcendence means experience beyond normal or common planes of existence. If you have awakened and have become a light worker and a star seed, then you are living a transcended life. Your frequency is elevated beyond that of a standard individual. You are living as an enlightened being.

If you have transcended, remember that everyone is at their own state of consciousness. Each of us understands, receives, and perceives information differently with diverse timing. Your frequency may become foreign to others if you have excelled further than them. Your elevated frequency can possibly make you feel like an outcast. Being ahead doesn't make you an outcast; it makes you a leader.

Aura – This form of the word aura means the energy field that radiates your personal vibration and frequency within and around you. This vibration reflects your purposes, moods, emotions, thoughts, and actions.

Your aura is within you and can extend to your personal surroundings. It interacts with your environments through any form of contact that you make with anyone or anything. Your spiritual aura operates within time space, yet isn't limited to it.

You can instantly have a noticeable auric shift by contact and interaction through something such as a text message. Even if the text was sent to or from someone centillions of miles away, the shift can be felt instantly. You could send someone on the other side of the world a letter in the mail, and as soon as they begin reading it, you may feel their frequency interacting with yours. You may also feel shifts as the letter passes through the possession of the carrier who delivers it. This is because you are able to feel the aura of the mail carrier as your frequency in your letter interacts with theirs. Your aura can interact with any action or reaction you cause anywhere.

Transverse – This form of the word transverse means situated or extending across something, like a bridgeway. (Mark 4:35)

The three dimensions are that which you live in, and the fourth dimension is anything outside of you. You are a being within a three-dimensional universe. The three dimensions are length, width, and height. Your body is your three-dimensional vessel. Anything outside of you is your fourth dimension. You could say that single men and women live in three-dimensional realities. Couples in relationships live in four-dimensional realities because their fourth dimension is their partner. Children are also their parent's fourth dimension.

The fifth dimension is the spiritual connection between your three dimensions and anything outside of you. The fifth dimension transverses the third and fourth dimensions. Because of the fifth dimension, you can feel the energy of others when they speak to you or even when they think about you. The fifth dimension bridges the gap between each of you and is part of the spirit realm.

Your aura transverses the physical and spiritual realms. Love builds a bridgeway for auras to interact. When you love someone, their aura can communicate with yours. When you send a text message or letter to someone, a traverse connection is built, allowing energetic transfers between you and them.

The goal here on Earth is to transverse the physical and spiritual realms. You can encounter GOD in every situation and in every moment. Learn to meet GOD within yourself first. Then you can express the light of GOD into the world from within your authenticity and love. This will help you transverse spirit with the physical realm.

Sleeping vs. Awakened

Sleeping vs. Awakened – These forms of these words, sleeping and awakened, mean the difference between consciously producing or unconsciously reacting. As it is currently, most people are in an action-reaction state, which is sometimes known as sleeping.

You are aligned into a precisely calculated experience that is prewritten. (Job 15:28) (Luke 2:34) (Romans 8:29-30) (Ephesians 1:5-11) Each person is a mathematical combination of action and reaction. Existence is viewed as it all happens within and around you. You are seamlessly a part of the universe.

If your experience enters a state where you decide to rewrite your script, then you have reactively come to that decision as part of your experience. You may believe that you have real free will. Your past experiences have programmed your mind to react by making certain decisions. Whenever something happens around you, there is a program within your mind and heart that tells you how to react. Your reaction is based on how your experiences have predetermined your response. Your cognitive and emotional psyche both interact similarly to the ways that elements in the periodic table react with one another.

How can this be?

We as people were initiated into our experiences through interactions with things such as our family and social dynamics. You have received your intellectual and physical codes of information from being part of those experiences. Within your environment, you continue to exchange codes and information with people, places, and things. The aspects of this world have integrated into you. Your experience is also coded into your DNA and neurological pathways. You are in the quantum field.

If this is true, then how do you use free will? Begin with the comprehension that sin doesn't actually exist. There is merely that which works and that which doesn't. Some things benefit, and others don't. Some ideas and paths help progression while others cannot.

Consider a planet in the terrestrial heavens. It has gravity that brings in a meteor and pulls it towards itself till it smashes against its own elements. Nature is similarly reactive and completely sinless altogether. People's personalities, wills, and intentions are like gravity, pulling in other people's personalities, wills, and intents. We collide and combine, like elements mixing together in chemistry. The colliding of personalities is like a fractal gravity. Some personalities and wills are not subject to the pull of particular personalities and intents, yet will be subject to others. Look at planets like Jupiter versus Earth. Planets too large can be physically violent and powerful, having so much forceful gravitational pull that it cannot sustain spiritual life on its surface. All things in the universe, including personalities, are designed like nature itself. Nature has no sin, and therefore people having been practiced upon the same natural platform of existence; we being harnessers of one another, are sinless.

A planet is born and then dies, eventually becoming something else. All of this is the natural perfected path of the process of nature. If it were a sin to drop a bomb, then it would be a sin for an asteroid to hit Jupiter. People's behaviors are natural fundamental reactions. All beings are systematically part of the process of nature, and their personalities, wills, and intents have guided each other's paths. What this means is that your decisions are not your own.

Humanity is a collective chemistry like the clouds on Jupiter. The entire universe is mathematically calculated to happen as it does, and your decisions and actions are a part of it all. You are a figment of reactive physics. Your experience is simply a view of it all happening.

If you can stand outside of this nature while inside of it, then you are within yet without. In spirituality, you can resist being empathically pulled into ways of degradation, so as not to allow forces to drag you anywhere they want. Then you are not only natural. You can put your delight into an intellectual rocket ship and propel from the social gravity that holds righteous ideas down.

So how do you exit this universal programming, also known as the matrix or the reactosphere? (Isaiah 49:1)

There is only one way to exit the formulaic expression that you are experiencing. Become spiritual. The Spirit is not limited to the equational process of the universe. Spirit isn't limited to the action-reaction state because Spirit isn't limited to linear time. The apparent evidence of this is found in the fact that incoming anger doesn't affect an advanced spiritual person. (Ephesians 4:3) The spiritual individual has the ability to remain calm through opposition.

Your placement in the reactosphere can be adjusted. GOD can help you reset your equation. (Ezra 3:5) The Spirit is alive. (Proverbs 20:27) GOD can shift the current equation within your mind, making sure that you are not a direct reflection of the action and reaction of your surroundings. Being with GOD can detach you from the action/reaction state of the existing seamlessness of the physical universe. GOD can adjust your mind to a place other than that which your upbringings and surroundings have placed you into. GOD will also allow you to do this within the Spirit.

You can wake up and step into your true position in life. People are feeling it now. Many are going to be making the transition towards purpose. They are entering the path that they originally signed up for so that they can fully anchor in the new Earth. What did you come here to do?

You may ask yourself, why would anyone want to wake up?

When you awaken, you can elevate your frequency within the Spirit, and anchor in your new energies. You can be supported and supportive in both the physical as well as the ethereal. When your vibration is spiritually solidified, you can then adjust the collective consciousness of humanity. Instead of you being a product of your environment, your environment becomes a product of you.

Your life is a pivotal point in time when your interaction with the community creates the ripple effect through everyone's reality. The result extends throughout this earthly experience. That is why your time and energy are so precious.

When you awaken more fully, you get a codex that holds information to be received for others around you. It is like a download of new information which causes a paradigm shift in the way you think and feel. When it happens, waking up is a beautiful and exciting journey.

At first, when you awaken, you may feel dislodged from your social surroundings. You may feel like you aren't part of the world anymore. (John 15:19, 16:33, 17:11-18, 18:36) (Romans 12:2) (1 Corinthians 2:14) (2 Corinthians 6:17) (1 Peter 2:9) (1 John 4:5, 5:19) Fear not. You have been called to a greater mission.

When you open your new path, you commence rewriting the experience that you are having. You begin reverse engineering your mind as you grow. You will begin opening space within your consciousness for new thought patterns. This allows you to learn vast new things and retrain your nervous system. You have the ability to create your experience, and that opens different possibilities for everyone. With your new comprehension, you can decide to rewrite the experience of all humanity.

Connect your natural and spiritual essences together. Secure your new growth and light into the future. Activate your energy and keep yourself very clear. You can make a meaningful impact just in the frequency of you being around someone. You can translate and transfer information energetically. The new energy that you share remains in the conscious collective.

You don't need to expect immediate results. Just getting your starseed into the people is enough. Implement the power of intention when planting starseeds for the future.

You are here to raise the vibration and frequency of the planet for humanity. Allow your vibration to be a product of your spiritual mind and heart, not just your environment. (1 John 2:5, 4:7-8) Live within the purpose that GOD has created for you. Be intentional with your attention. It will be exciting receiving all the codes and love that you open. (Ephesians 3:14-19)

Being awakened has sometimes been known as becoming a Buddha, or, in other words, an awakened one. Know that everyone chooses different levels of how far they want to grow. Not everyone wants to wake up. Sleep is comforting and sweet to many of them. (Jeremiah 31:26) Some people may never wake up. Those who sleep are considered elements of reactive nature. (Jeremiah 51:39, 51:57)

If you have read this explanation on sleeping vs. awakened, know that the explanation of sin not existing doesn't mean that you can do anything that you want and still live in the Spirit of GOD. There is a forbidden fruit, and we are warned not to eat from it. You can find an explanation in Chapter 8 of this book.

Quantum Leap – This term means an awakening leading to an abrupt transition in your life. Some people go through sudden and often unexpected transitions when they wake up spiritually, and their life becomes temporarily unmanageable. This can also be called quantum shifting or quantum jumping.

We as people evolve over time. You may not want to change, yet some changes are very good for you. It is ok for you to make way for the new. It is helpful to embrace the beauty of transformation. This book is for assisting your alignment to the greatest frequencies that our ancestors were attempting to evolve towards.

Humanity is in a pivotal moment. The collective frequency is shifting through a quantum leap. The world is rearranging, and you may feel the changes. These experiences are taking place so that you can see and choose your path. Humanity is stepping away from one reality and into another.

Are you here to serve a greater mission? Do you feel in your essence and being that there is something important that you are supposed to do? Even if you don't have full clarity of what it is yet, rely on GOD to guide you through the process.

We are opening and increasing ourselves when we choose to evolve, grow, and change. You are presented with choices and opportunities to decide upon a greater evolutionary growth. What will you choose?

Your abilities are possible to achieve. You have a chance to adopt the elevated alignment that you have been searching for. Implement your chosen level of shift into reality, and be reborn as a new being. (John 3:3-8) (1 Peter 1:22-23)

When you are reborn into a new state of consciousness, you will attract different experiences. You will have greater insight. Focus on stabilizing your new frequency until you are fully acclimated to your new vibration. As you increase your frequency, the vibration in your cells, molecules, and atoms will also increase.

You may feel like you have found a new identity, a new you. If you have shifted, the way you view the experience that you are having will have changed with it. You may have had a quantum leap, also known as waking up.

You may be feeling an urgency inside of you, that you did a quantum leap and touched a greater state of consciousness. You may have reached new energies and frequencies. If so, a new life is now possible with what has opened for you. You will begin making decisions from a reborn consciousness. You will have a different synapse in your mind, with different cognitive and emotional ideas for making decisions. Enter the ways of the greater frequencies that you choose to obtain.

You have a chance to help usher in the new heaven and the new Earth. (Isaiah 66:22) You are the journey. Your thoughts shape your reality. You can send your energetic shifts throughout humanity. When you solidify your new energetics, anchoring them into your surroundings, even the entirety of the cosmos feels the impact of your expanse.

When you awaken, you get to decide where you will land. You can progress in as many stages as you choose. You may choose one step, or even to increase within yourself to the fullest capacity. You get to input the plane of your energetic improvement into the collective consciousness.

Know this: when you increase, not everyone around you will be on the same level. Different people will be in different stages of consciousness. Not everyone comprehends every intensity yet.

Akashic Records – The Akashic Records are recordings of each individual's existence, from the creation of their spirit onward. These records include your experience(s) and all your memories. Your Akashic Record is also known as your soul. Everything that you have been and all that you have done is recorded there.

Divine Blueprint – This term means the personality and purpose of your spirit when GOD first created your Akashic record. Your divine blueprint was GOD's original creation plan for you. This is also known as your spirit or true personality.

Before your incarnation here, you signed up for the lessons that you wanted to learn. You were input into a physical experience within this three-dimensional matter wherever you and GOD chose for you to enter. There are many other spirits peering through matter into existence. While here, the ways of others can shift you away from your original creation plan and path.

The work in the Akashic Records is to connect you to your divine blueprint. This means to reconnect your soul (memory) to your spirit (true personality). Your original blueprint (spirit) is your original frequency and your original plan. As you experience this world, your path and frequency are adjusted through contact with people, places, and things. As we live, we can grow further from our original divine blueprint. Accessing the Akashic Records helps realign us to the individual original plan that we had before we were even born.

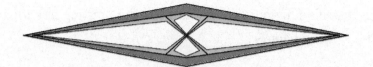

Chapter 2
Planting Starseeds – Ora's Starseed

This chapter is a continuance from chapter one. It focuses more on the practices and purposes of lightworkers and starseeds.

Meditate – This form of the word meditation means to think deeply and focus. Though you can meditate at any time, anywhere, and during any day, even in a noisy environment, meditation is best when done in peaceful silence.

We can each have a spiritual journey. By accessing your Akashic Records through meditation, you have the possibility to reconnect your potentials to your divine blueprint. You can restore your future by realigning your position in life to GOD's original plan for you. Align yourself to GOD's will and tune into Divine Source. This will help you achieve a desirable outcome during your experience. It will also help your life become beneficial to everyone.

Your interactions can lead you away from your true essence. When you meditate, clear yourself of external interruptions, including noise, stimuli, and outer interferences. Detach from accumulated debris so that you can claim remembrance of who you really are in the essence of your wholeness. Tune into your connection with GOD. You may be much more than you have ever realized. Consider your goals. What was your purpose to begin with? Rediscover the real you, and activate your divine blueprint through meditation.

Divine Intuition – This term means your ability to spiritually discern based on promptings from the Spirit, Holy Ghost, and Holy Spirit. Divine intuition can help you sense things within the quantum field from a spiritual perspective.

Meditations can be used to learn how to listen to the energies within the quantum field. While in a calm state with your eyes closed, you may see, hear, smell, taste, and feel things both physically and spiritually. These particular sensations are not always from the physical realm. They are often sensed within your divine intuition. You can practice listening to your divine intuition while resting or sitting in a meditative position. Some people also meditate while in nature.

For many people, divine intuition can be sensed in a vision while laying down as if going to sleep. It helps if you are not overly tired. During the moment of hypnagogia while dozing off and in hypnopompia while waking up, a picture may flash before your eyes. You may also hear a voice. These types of visions can be used as guidance. Be careful because these visions usually need translating to find the meaning. Conventional translations are often incorrect. You will have to learn what they mean through experience.

Accept your intuition as guidance towards what feels authentic and true to you. You may incur visions that push you to grow. This can help make your pathways clear so that you can see better. One example is that your intuition reveals a picture of something that you are being told to do. If you know that your intuition is telling you to do something wrong, then resist what it is telling you to do. It isn't actually your intuition misguiding you. This is your intuitive ability to build resistance to any opposition to your authenticity.

When you meditate, you can enter a calm space where you can listen to your intuition. It should lead you to seek GOD's divine guidance. With GOD's direction, you can see the path that you should be on. (Psalm 77:12, 119:15, 119:27, 119:48, 119:148, 145:5) (Philippians 4:8) (1 Timothy 4:15) Once you are being divinely guided, see that each part of your life is contributing to where you want to go. Focus on something good that serves your purpose with GOD, something that will propel you forward in life. Everything is working towards your benefit. Trust that all things are lining up for success. You are worthy.

When you learn to cultivate intuitive guidance in conjunction with divine intuition, you can see things from a greater perspective. Close your eyes and just anchor into your peacefulness. Know that everything is fine.

Using your Spiritual Vessel for Conscious Navigation – This idea means to intentionally navigate through life by spiritually tuning your body into a purposeful awakened consciousness. (1 Corinthians 15:44)

There are many ways to consciously navigate through life. This is about finding your path by connecting your spirituality with your body. Have you cultivated a connection between the vessel that you live in and the Spirit? Your body holds wisdom, and you can use it as a navigation system. Your spirit and body can be tuned together to help you make choices. You can use spiritual and physical feelings to help direct your decisions.

Here is a meditative practice designed to help you learn how.

First, enter your calm, central self. While within your inner peace, ask your body to show you what 'yes' feels like. Notice any sensations that you feel when you say yes. Notice any impressions in your stomach. Does anything feel lighter in your body when you ask about yes and acceptance? Do you sense anything within your vessel?

Now clear that and recenter with a deep breath. Next, ask your body to show you what 'no' feels like. Notice any sensations that you feel when you say no. Notice any impressions in your stomach. Does anything feel heavier in your body when you ask about no and denial? Is there a sensation within your vessel? Breathe a few deep breaths and notice if and where you feel tension in your body. You may sense tightness somewhere, such as in your stomach. Even the slightest minute shift in energy may be noticed. Everyone is different, so whatever you feel is for you. (2 Corinthians 1:17-19) (James 5:12)

The way you use your navigation system is personal to what you are and what you have activated. This technique can help you when making choices. Tune into your inner peace and ask yourself how you will feel about the outcome before you decide something. This can help keep your decisions in alignment with your greatest timeline. You can ask if your decision is in alignment with your best path. You may need to practice tuning into feeling the sensations. This is an exercise for intuitive guidance.

When practicing this, a lighter feeling means free and energetically filled. A heavier feeling means draining and locked down. Using light and heavy feelings to direct your way through navigation is a feminine aspect. However, the masculine aspect uses logic to discover and explain why something is. You need both masculine and feminine when making good decisions. Your feminine aspect alone would always agree to engage in the lighter feeling energies. Lighter feelings are the energies that feel good to be around. They comfort you. Sometimes that comfort can be a trap, and logic explains why.

It is common for people practicing energetics to go in the direction that feels the best. It has been said that energy doesn't lie. The laws of physics are designed in a way that can look like a lie. For instance, the Earth can seem flat until you look at it while standing on the moon. Depending on where you view something from, the perception can change. There are countless illusions that can be demonstrated.

Imagine children at home while their parents are at work. There is a cookie jar on the counter, and they are not allowed to have a treat yet. One child knows that the parents won't find out who took a cookie if one is eaten. Since there are several children and no parents observing, one child takes a cookie and eats it. Since the parents are at work, the child can lie and not be known. If the parents were home, and the children were being observed, then the child wouldn't take the cookie knowing that the parents would see.

Likewise in the quantum field, we have at least one observation where energy does something different when it is being watched. In the double-slit experiment where electrons or photons are passed through two slits, the results are different when the energy is being observed. This outcome reveals that energy is like a child with a cookie jar. Here are a couple of links that reveal this quantum research.

https://youtu.be/ZQAvVgnreWk

https://youtu.be/5kfGRO6msQw

Though in many forms it is true that energy doesn't lie, it can also be like candy. Sugar may feel good on your tongue, yet it can also rot your teeth out. Be careful with that perfect-feeling energy. Just like sugar tastes good, comforting energy can be used to honor deceitfulness and incorrect paths. Sometimes the energy that doesn't feel so good is the energy that you need to face so that you can grow.

While a heavy energy can drain you or make you feel locked down, heavy can also be correct. Sometimes that heavy energy is there to reveal that which is draining you and locking you down in the first place. Instead of running from energies that hold a heaviness, learn to logicize why the energy is heavy. Use your masculine as well as your feminine. The masculine can be used in the quantum field to explain reasonings based on scientific fact and example.

Imagine a group of people who constantly relax and eat tasty junk food. They then began to have muscle atrophy and heart problems. These people soon go to the doctor for medical help. The doctor offers two options for the patients. The first option is medication, which can treat the symptom without helping the problem. The medication is an easy path that isn't heavy. Easy gives them a good feeling. They can then use the drug and remain relaxed and unhealthy. The second option is that the doctor helps them treat the actual problem instead of the symptom. The doctor prescribes exercise several days per week, possibly at a gym, and advises them to eat healthier food. That answer may feel very heavy to the patients. Because of this, the patients may ignore the solution and opt to treat the symptoms instead. They may even skip the exercise and enjoy the comfort of a massage chair. That heavy feeling energy represents the problem being locked down.

Here is another example of moments that you must use logic to interpret your energetic feelings. Imagine that two people met and began a relationship. Suddenly, one of them got an uncomfortable sensation about their new partner. Feelings like these could be from an outside friend or family member. Your aura is connected and merged to those that you are close to. Sometimes your feelings about someone are issues of acceptance within your social connections. Your close relations can help decide things for you when their aura is merged with yours. This is because the frequencies of your close companions are transversed into you. Their vibrations, being within you, may reject the vibrations of someone else. When this happens, you must use logic to see what they don't want that person for. It is very common for people who are sleeping in a state of comfortableness to reject something productive and purposeful. Social groups often want everyone to remain where they are. Close comrades may have a tendency to want you in a station that benefits their position instead of your own. Evolution is frequently rejected by those who don't want change.

It isn't always fun to choose the form of energy that helps you grow. Sometimes the energy that doesn't feel as good is exactly what you really need. This is like going to the gym. To build muscle, you must exert the muscles so that they can grow. This is the same in the quantum field of energetics. Sometimes that which doesn't immediately feel as good happens to be the future of bettering your quantum health.

Some heavy-feeling energies are good, and others are unsafe. Being able to define which heavy feelings are good for you is important. If it is heavy because of the wills of others, then the heaviness warns of their intentions for you. If it is heavy because you don't want to stimulate growth by exiting your comfort zone, then the heaviness is a warning of how you limit yourself. Knowing these facts can help you determine whether or not a heavy energy is harmful or helpful.

Conscious Elemental Interaction – This idea is about your ability to consciously interact with the elements and the universe. You can shift the vibrations of the elements.

You may become very educated in using your body as a navigation system. There are many ways that you can sense with your vessel. Consider water, for example. Your emotions, thoughts, and actions are held within the vibrations of the water within you. The water communicates through these vibrations.

Contemplate the experiments that Dr. Emoto did on water. He changed the molecular structure of water by interacting with it through emotions, intentions, and sounds. According to him, speaking to water using words infused with emotions and intent before freezing it had affected the shape of the ice crystals. When he spoke rude or derogative words to the water, the ice crystals would then be misshapen. When he spoke encouraging and loving words to the water, the ice crystals would be attractive and symmetric like artistic snowflakes. With symmetry is strength and stability.

Some people can read emotions through water. They can sense the water's vibrations. Water communicates through their system, causing them to be able to sense the frequencies within another person. It is believed that showing gratitude to the water and being thankful can code those vibrations into it.

Your body may be as much as 60% water or more. The emotions that radiate through your body affect the water molecules within you. Being happy and loving produces stability. Anger can cause a decline in health.

People who get mad become unstable and destructive to themselves and their surroundings. It is important to create healing frequencies within you, that they radiate throughout you and your surroundings.

By integrating a new belief system into who you are, that system's frequencies enter your cells, molecules, and atoms. Practicing gratitude and kindness can boost your immune system and enhance the law of attraction. Acknowledge and focus on the things that are going correctly in your life. Recognize that everything is working towards the good. This will shift your reality. Notice that GOD works through you to create something different in this experience.

According to some people, water has wisdom and healing gifts that you can utilize. You can communicate with the water freely. You can ask the water to cleanse your auric field. You can speak to the water within you, asking it to flush and cleanse your system to remove toxins and impurities that are not beneficial. Some say that while bathing, you can receive information from the water in pictures or words, or that you can feel information in a knowing through meditation. That is very dependent on how you read energy. Ask GOD what any information you receive means.

You can communicate with each of the elements that your spirit lives within. Be at peace with the water, the oxygen, the iron, and all the elements that facilitate your quantum experience. Every element and the entire universe can feel your energy. When using this practice, it is important to remember that the LORD is beyond all matter. While the LORD can be within all things, GOD is also beyond definition. Be careful before considering an elemental vibration to be a message from GOD. (1 Kings 19:10-13) We will always learn from the LORD.

Energetic Shields – This idea is about putting up energetic shields that can help protect you from certain energies, vibrations, and frequencies.

It is a common belief that once you are in tune with feeling vibrations and frequencies, you can program your auric energy field. Here is a meditative practice that you can use to do this.

Close your eyes. Breathe in through your nose, and imagine the energy filling you from your toes to the top of your head. When you get a nice deep breath that fills your lungs, hold it in. Then release it through your mouth. Breathe in and out like this three times. Take notice of any thoughts that you have. Find your inner peace. If you have judgments, or if you are trying to overanalyze, just let that go as you do this. Anchor more fully into your essence. Feel your own energy without all that noise and chatter that comes from the mind or anything that you may have picked up from other people. Release all of that. Inhale deeply.

Keep your eyes closed while you sense the energy of your auric field. Tune in. What does the energy that runs along your body feel like? Focus on that for a moment, and expand it outward by using your imagination to see it. Notice how far you can expand the energy field. It is ok if you don't entirely feel anything. Something is happening. While meditating, what is a color, symbol, frequency, or sensation that comes up for you around the thought of protection? Whatever you sense when you focus on the word protection should be something that can assist you in programming your energy field. Ask GOD what it means.

Visualize and put helpful, intuitive frequencies into your energetic path. Within your intention, state what you want the protection to deflect. You can visualize it all around you if that helps. You can tune it to deflect anything not in alignment with your best path, only allowing love and the logical frequencies that you want and need. You will learn to protect, trust, and hear yourself more. Ask GOD to help you through the process. This can also guide you in learning to listen to GOD better.

Lightworkers – This form of the word lightworkers means those who work to help others find and succeed in their beneficial purposes and missions. They help people achieve divine assignments. They work to raise the vibration of humanity. They also help the health of the earth and various types of environments. They bring light to situations. They offer good energies, frequencies, vibrations, knowledge, intellect, wisdom, emotions, and anything else that can help.

To be a lightworker, you must first activate the light of your divine assignment. There are four main stages to turning on your light. Each step is important.

1: Begin with the comprehension that you are a spirit being, and your physical body is your garment. Cleanse away anything that has kept you separated from the DIVINE. Acknowledge the CREATOR. Pray and forgive others. Hold no resentment, and put your trust in GOD. Your physical vessel will be able to hold much more light when you cultivate your connection with GOD.

2: In order to connect to SOURCE, you must increase your capacity for spiritual light through personal cleansing. Possibly the most important instrument for cleansing your aura is honesty with yourself and others. Meditation can also help with this.

3: Cast out selfishness and freely help others in any way you can. Giving is an important factor in activating your light. Random acts of kindness and generosity without expecting anything in return from others is how this is done. This is called doing spiritual works. Any deed done that requires money or items in return isn't a spiritual deed. GOD doesn't recognize spirituality done in exchange for money. (Matthew 10:8) (1 Corinthians 2:12) (2 Corinthians 8:3) (Revelation 21:6, 22:17)

4: Anchor helpful behaviors into your body and daily life. Focus on being a clean and efficient being. Operating this way will raise your vibration. This means that you must be consciously considering and doing things such as recycling and using fuel-efficient methods of transportation. Refrain from taking more in life than one person needs. Doing your best to be efficient means that you are not carelessly taking from others. Everything you save is being saved for all of humanity.

Once you have cleansed and activated your light, you can then do lightwork. Lightwork is the process of extending your light beyond your own physical vessel. When doing lightwork, comprehend that you are a spirit being. Now see that the entire universe is your garment. You can traverse your light into everyone and everything through unification with your monadic self.

Examples of ways to extend your light are simple, such as smiling and sharing gratitude. Be thankful. Direct your light into everything around you. Be optimistic when conversing. Everything you do can be beneficial and healing. Your actions will prompt good outcomes. Also, your frequency, since it is enlightened, will increase the light in everything that you interact with.

Those who want to usher in the new era of the elevated caliber of existence are choosing transcendence and connecting with GOD. We find in the ancient Gnostics that the perfected being is connected to GOD who is the monad source of all. You may find it helpful to seek silence through meditation when connecting to the SOURCE FREQUENCY. Doing this can assist in you becoming a new you.

Here are some Gnostic quotes that examine ancient clues about connecting to GOD and turning on your light. These can be helpful depending on how you perceive them.

(Gnostic The Apocryphon of John) "Now, therefore, lift up your face, that you may receive the things that I shall teach you today, and may tell them to your fellow spirits who are from the unwavering race of the perfect Man." And I asked to know it, and he said to me, "The Monad is a monarchy with nothing above it. It is he who exists as God and Father of everything, the invisible One who is above everything, who exists as incorruption, which is in the pure light into which no eye can look."

CODEX II Translated by Frederik Wisse Selection made from James M. Robinson, ed., The Nag Hammadi Library, revised edition. HarperCollins, San Francisco, 1990.

(Gnostic The Second Treatise of the Great Seth) "They stand ready to receive the life-giving word of the ineffable Monad and of the greatness of the assembly of all those who persevere and those who are in me. I visited a bodily dwelling. I cast out the one who was in it first, and I went in. And the whole multitude of the archons became troubled. And all the matter of the archons, as well as all the begotten powers of the earth, were shaken when it saw the likeness of the Image, since it was mixed. And I am the one who was in it, not resembling him who was in it first. For he was an earthly man, but I, I am from above the heavens. I did not refuse them even to become a Christ, but I did not reveal myself to them in the love which was coming forth from me. I revealed that I am a stranger to the regions below. There was a great disturbance in the whole earthly area, with confusion and flight, as well as (in) the plan of the archons. And some were persuaded, when they saw the wonders which were being accomplished by me. And all these, with the race, that came down, flee from him who had fled from the throne to the Sophia of hope, since she had earlier given the sign concerning us and all the ones with me - those of the race of Adonaios."

(Gnostic The Second Treatise of the Great Seth) "And surrounding him, he appears to him as a Monad of all these, a thought and a father, since he is one. And he stands by them all, since he as a whole came forth alone. And he is life, since he came from the Father of ineffable and perfect Truth, (the father) of those who are there, the union of Peace and a friend of good things, and life eternal and undefiled joy, in a great harmony of life and faith, through eternal life of fatherhood and motherhood and sisterhood and rational wisdom."

CODEX VII Translated by Roger A. Bullard and Joseph A. Gibbons Selection made from James M. Robinson, ed., The Nag Hammadi Library, revised edition. HarperCollins, San Francisco, 1990.

(Gnostic The Valentinian Exposition) "Moreover it is these who have known him who is, the Father, that is, the Root of the All, the Ineffable One who dwells in the Monad. He dwells alone in silence, and silence is tranquility since, after all, he was a Monad and no one was before him. He dwells in the Dyad and in the Pair, and his Pair is Silence. And he possessed the All dwelling within him. And as for Intention and Persistence, Love and Permanence, they are indeed unbegotten. God came forth: the Son, Mind of the All, that is, it is from the Root of the All that even his Thought stems, since he had this one (the Son) in Mind. For on behalf of the All, he received an alien Thought since there were nothing before him. From that place it is he who moved [...] a gushing spring. Now this is the Root of the All and Monad without any one before him. Now the second spring exists in silence and speaks with him alone."

CODEX XI Translated by John D. Turner Selection made from James M. Robinson, ed., The Nag Hammadi Library, revised edition. HarperCollins, San Francisco, 1990.

(Gnostic The Second Apocalypse of James) "And they follow you; they enter and you escort them inside, and give a reward to each one who is ready for it. For you are not the redeemer nor a helper of strangers. You are an illuminator and a redeemer of those who are mine, and now of those who are yours. You shall reveal (to them); you shall bring good among them all."

CODEX V Translated by Charles W. Hedrick Selection made from James M. Robinson, ed., The Nag Hammadi Library, revised edition. HarperCollins, San Francisco, 1990.

(Gnostic Apocalypse of Adam) "This is the hidden knowledge of Adam, which he gave to Seth, which is the holy baptism of those who know the eternal knowledge through those born of the word and the imperishable illuminators, who came from the holy seed: Yesseus, Mazareus, Yessedekeus, the Living Water."

CODEX V Translated by George W. MacRae Selection made from James M. Robinson, ed., The Nag Hammadi Library, revised edition. HarperCollins, San Francisco, 1990.

(Gnostic The Prayer of Thanksgiving) "We rejoice, having been illuminated by Your knowledge. We rejoice because You have shown us Yourself. We rejoice because while we were in (the) body, You have made us divine through Your knowledge. "The thanksgiving of the man who attains to You is one thing: that we know You. We have known You, intellectual light. Life of life, we have known You. Womb of every creature, we have known You. Womb pregnant with the nature of the Father, we have known You."

CODEX VI Translated by James Brashler, Peter A. Dirkse and Douglas M. Parrott Selection made from James M. Robinson, ed., The Nag Hammadi Library, revised edition. HarperCollins, San Francisco, 1990.

(Gnostic The Teachings of Sylvanus) "Did you (fem. sg.) wish to become animal when you had come into this kind of nature? But rather, share in a true nature of life. To be sure, animality will guide you into the race of the earth, but the rational nature will guide you in rational ways. Turn toward the rational nature, and cast from yourself the earth-begotten nature. O soul, persistent one, be sober and shake off your drunkenness, which is the work of ignorance. If you persist and live in the body, you dwell in rusticity. When you entered into a bodily birth, you were begotten. Come into being inside the bridal chamber! Be illuminated in mind!"

(Gnostic The Teachings of Sylvanus) "Live with Christ and he will save you. For he is the true light and the sun of life. For just as the sun which is visible and makes light for the eyes of the flesh, so Christ illuminates every mind and the heart."

CODEX VII Translated by Malcolm L. Peel and Jan Zandee Selection made from James M. Robinson, ed., The Nag Hammadi Library, revised edition. HarperCollins, San Francisco, 1990.

(Gnostic The Letter of Peter to Philip) "When you strip off from yourselves what is corrupted, then you will become illuminators in the midst of mortal men.""

CODEX VIII Translated by Frederik Wisse Selection made from James M. Robinson, ed., The Nag Hammadi Library, revised edition. HarperCollins, San Francisco, 1990.

Avatar – This form of the word avatar means a being that is transversed between two places or realms.

You are a spirit being who exists within the spirit realm. Your spirit enters the physical realm as an avatar and experiences a physical life.

Another form of avatar is when you are an extraterrestrial being in the terrestrial heaven while also living within a human body. This second form of avatar happens when an extraterrestrial (Angel) sends your soul into a body by using a signal. Avatars are sent information and are controlled from above. Their actual thought processes happen on the other side of their veils and are sent into them. The extraterrestrial angel is the primary life, and the avatar is the secondary life.

Starseed – This form of the word starseed means a lightworker's illuminated inner light, which can be planted into the conscious collective of humanity Planting your starseed is part of your lightwork. Your starseed can include an accumulation of your works.

It is said that starseeds are people who came from another place. Many people believe that their soul originated from a distant planet, galaxy, universe, or dimension. According to them, their first life or lives were somewhere else, and they were later incarnated here on Earth.

It isn't impossible for you to have lived somewhere else. There are two known ways for this to occur. The first way that this can happen is if GOD has appointed for you to be incarnated or reincarnated on Earth after a previous life.

1: GOD may have a plan for you to do something here on Earth, even if you didn't live here first. Your spirit could have been sent here by GOD into a new physical body. When this happens, your spirit being is sent to earth, and your entire soul recording is in the spiritual realm.

2: Your soul can be recorded by the angels in this realm. These angels are extraterrestrial beings that have the ability to travel between solar systems and galaxies. They use things like semisynthetic-biological computers to record your soul as you live. They can then plant your soul recording into another body through signals. These signals are more advanced than radio waves and can penetrate any body. These extraterrestrials have ships that they can live in. When they plant a soul into someone, the host becomes an avatar. The avatar doesn't always remember any past lives. This is because of the one-way veil put between the harborer's ship and the host. As an avatar, you are a conscious harborer in the ship. You can see your host body, yet from within your host body you cannot always see your other side. The host isn't in any physical danger when they become an avatar. It is like the host is a puppet that the harborer lives within. The harborer controls the host and experiences the host's life as if being in a virtual reality system. When you leave your body here on earth, you remain on your ship. You can then be reinput into another body. These angels are tremendously advanced. They have rules and regulations through covenants. They don't usually just take any body they want at any time without good reason. Angels usually avatar a body before the age of two.

Regardless of however many lives you may have lived in however many places, your soul (akashic record) originated from GOD. Your spirit (divine blueprint) also originated from GOD. In order for your starseed to survive, it must be tuned into your true origin.

The Tao, known as the Mother of All things, means GOD in feminine form. SHE is the SOURCE form of the HOLY GHOST. She is also known as WISDOM. (Proverbs 8:12-36) (Wisdom 7:7, 7:22-24)

(Tao Te Ching 1) "(Conceived of as) having no name, it is the Originator of heaven and earth; (conceived of as) having a name, it is the Mother of all things."

By Lao Tzu. Translated by J. Legge 1891.

Wherever you have been and whoever you are, remember that your only true source origin is GOD. If you have traveled here from another place, you must be tuned into the SOURCE ORIGIN for your mission to be found worthy. GOD's agenda is always acceptable. Even if you are from another planet, your path must be along GOD's agenda. Your true source origin is GOD.

You can be a starseed even if this is your first life. Starseed doesn't just mean that you came from somewhere else. Your starseed is something beneficial that you are planting here on Earth which has been sourced from another place or plane or existence.

We know that Abraham was told that his children would be as the stars of heaven. (Exodus 32:13) Abraham's children connect to GOD as their source origin. This is the most important part of planting your starseed. Even if you are not a literal descendant of Abraham, you can be adopted as a child of GOD through his covenant. (Romans 8:15, 8:23) (Galatians 4:5, 4:28) (Ephesians 1:5) (Hebrews 11:18)

In order for your starseed to grow after being planted, you must be tuned to Divine Source. Your mission is about turning people to righteousness. (Daniel 12:3) Tune to GOD.

Those doing lightwork have cleansed their frequency and activated their light. Once your light is turned on, it can be planted as a seed. You can sow your frequency into the conscious collective of humanity. Doing this raises the vibrational energy within the people. Your frequency is also planted into the mainframe of the cosmos. Whatever you plant should be an acceptable offering.

As a lightworker, your goal is to have a helpful seed that can be safely sown. Healthy ideas, intentions, and actions are the strength of a good starseed. Well-established starseeds help everyone. Good deeds and frequencies are contagious.

You will need a place to deep seat your light roots, and there are many ways to seal your frequency into the people. This is where you must choose the path that you will travel on. What type of frequency elevation will you offer? What light job will you choose? You can feed the needy. You can write a helpful book. You can do Reiki. You can even give hugs to random people. Just as the common saying that smiles are contagious, an illuminated frequency can also be transmitted. You can merge your vibration each time you come into contact with someone. There are countless options. Remember that whatever you do to transfer and plant your starseed must be done freely without charge.

Once sewn, your starseed needs to be watered and nurtured so it may grow. In order for your starseed to be watered after being planted, you must be tuned to Divine Source. Your mission is to bring people towards righteousness. (Daniel 12:3) If your idea is tuned to GOD, then GOD will ensure that your seed is watered. (1 Corinthians 3:5-17) Amplify your manifestation and light the pathway for others.

You are employed to anchor in a new vibration. This doctrine is offered to help set in a new energy. You can integrate your personal information with what you learn. This book is aligned to Source Frequency and the evolved vibration of your greatest timeline. You can recalibrate your frequency by using this path. A new energy will help you make better choices and will draw others towards you. They will reciprocate that which you are putting out. The greater level of choices you make, the better reflection that others will return in your favor. You initiate the harmony that you live in.

When you clear up your energetics, it also cleanses your DNA. By doing the cleansing work, you are changed on a molecular level. This alters the frequency in your atoms, DNA, and molecules. When you raise your energetic vibration, you also help realign the path of your family lineage. This happens because your aura encompasses your children. It can even extend into your close relatives and into their children for those who don't have their own.

You are in a wonderful position in life. You get to set the tone for the future of your descendants and for all humanity. Your energy is important, and you are needed. Anchor your frequency into the people. You are to be celebrated as an important being.

The entire first and second chapters of this book were aligned with a starseed from Ora. She is a very educated Soul Coach who works in the quantum field. Ora's data was found to be important for everyone. She was also proven to have been called by GOD to deliver the information for this purpose. Because of this, her information was gathered and organized. The seed of Abraham was then planted into it. To do this, Ora's information was divinely aligned to source frequency through the Abrahamic covenant. When a man and woman merge their starseeds together, the woman's information becomes the lightwomb. The covenant seed aligned with Ora's information is a spiritual child. This is Ora's spiritual child of Abraham. (Luke 1:55) (Acts 3:25) (Exodus 32:13)

Soul Tribe or Soul Family – This term means two or more people that have similar energies, vibrations, and frequencies who can interact and grow well together. When they match and merge, their light increases.

When you have recalibrated your frequency to the greater path, you can plant your starseed. One way that you can do this is by anchoring your energy into your soul tribe. Securing your developed frequency into the people creates a ripple effect throughout the conscious collective.

Like you, each person has a specific and unique vibration. To locate your soul tribe, find people who are encouraging and inspiring towards you. If they meet your frequency, and if it feels correct, reflect on that. Find relationships that are solid and real. Those who reciprocate with you and increase your abilities are your soul family. Those who harness you and hold you down are not your soul family.

Your soul family may be a religious group. If you were to enter a religious assembly, and their vibrations matched yours, then they may be your soul tribe. This has been explained in different ways by many people, such as Christians. A Christian may enter several churches before they find one that feels aligned to their spirit. That is often how people find their correct religious home.

Quantum Entanglement – This term means the process of two or more perceptions, people, places, or things becoming united as if they are one.

Here are some explanations of various types of quantum entanglement.

Begin with learning about the ego-self. In the quantum field, there is an ego-self duality. There is a lower ego and a higher ego.

Singularity is the path of the lower ego. The lower ego is the self, which protects itself as itself. Your lower ego-self is the side of you that strives to be the best one, the one to trust, the one to go to, the best friend, and so on. The lower ego wants to harness and control others, grab life, and own it, hold onto possessions, etc. In the lower ego, people want to be themselves, and so they may avoid genuinely connecting to others. It wants itself to be the one that it has.

Unity is the path of the higher ego. The higher ego is the we, which protects ourselves as an us. Your higher ego is the side of you that strives to be there for others, to trust others, to go to others for help, seeks friends, and so on. The higher ego helps others be in control, helps them grab life and own it, willingly gives possessions without need of recognition, etc. In the higher ego, people want to be together, and so they seek genuine connections with others. It wants us to be the ones that we have.

There is a process that helps healthy merging of the lower and higher egos. This process will be examined as a relationship between man and woman. Watch, step by step, how the lower and higher egos enter quantum entanglement together.

The lower ego is the place for personal spirituality. In the lower ego, you have the chance to reflect upon yourself, consider your own ways, and build a personal relationship with GOD.

The process of becoming spiritual includes cleansing your lower ego of toxic debris. Become comfortable with who you are by developing what you desire in a partner. Live life in peace, not worrying about how each moment will go your way. Let go of attachments to unneeded control. Single out your own personal energy field and remove unhealthy bonds that may have merged with you and entered your aura. You can seek GOD's advice through meditation and prayer. Become something that you really like. Once you are cleansed, you then have yourself as a single being with a clean auric vibration.

To be ready to merge with and cleanse your higher ego-self, you must first cleanse your own personal being. This is where the saying, "you must love yourself before you can love another," comes from. You don't want to merge as a toxic addon. Once you have cleansed yourself and have founded a solid relationship with GOD, you must anchor your good path. Good wills, intentions, and behaviors should be solidified in your lower ego before entering the higher ego.

The next step is to let go of ego attachment to the self. Enter and merge into a relationship with one another. You must remember the lower ego cleansing that you don't attempt to force control of your companion. You will be willingly giving your partner authority over portions of your being. This reflects both ways.

Remember that you each remain the owner of the control that you offer. Lovers always share influence of one another in certain aspects. This sway is by consent. Each of you is blessed with the fact that your lover chose to share his or her life with you, yet you don't own one another. This fact keeps the relationship sacred. Either one of you has the choice to depart at any moment. The daily choice to remain together means that every day is special.

Now this is where the egos entangle. Your lower ego is the micro ego of yourself. Your higher ego is the macro-unified ego that you have together. When these two types of egos quantum entangle and merge in dual polarities, they are canceled out. This happens in true love when you refrain from taking control and receive the authority that your partner offers. Neither forces, yet both willingly give sway to one another. The lower and higher egos withdraw.

If you have cleansed your lower ego-self, then you can successfully cleanse your higher ego unity. (Matthew 7:5) (Luke 6:42) If you notice something toxic entering the relationship, you can take control of the situation. Does that mean that you are egotistical or that your lower ego is in control? When ego attachment to the self is used to protect the collective higher ego, the lower ego is then using a higher ego consciousness. This is why it is important to cleanse the lower ego and solidify good wills, intentions, and behaviors into yourself. Anchoring a healthy lower ego is required. When you hold onto your own beneficial ways, even against unhealthy opposition, you protect the collective. Therefore, the lower ego becomes a part of the higher ego consciousness.

Attachment to yourself when in the higher ego can actually be for protecting the collective. This means that anchoring the lower ego is a necessity. When you hold onto your own righteous ways to protect the collective, even against opposition, you reinforce safety in the unity. (2 Timothy 2:21-26) Therefore the lower ego is a part of the higher ego consciousness.

A lover that likes to be guided by his or her partner is evidence of a cleansed higher ego. Fundamental love doesn't need attachment to material possessions and control of worldly affairs. Lovers first gain and cleanse themselves in their lower ego and then share that ego control with their partner. Within the ego duality of true love, these two types of egos neutralize each other. The lower and higher egos quantum entangle, canceling each other out. Ego no longer exists as long as both the lower and higher selves remain intact. That which isn't is also that which is.

Cleansing yourself is done in the lower ego and must happen properly before you can safely entangle. Quantum entanglement into the fourth and fifth dimensions is the higher ego. Trust your masculine and feminine communications because each one is the other required half of the frequency field. Health comes from both polarities being perfectly united.

If you got hurt, would your partner be able to reflect his or her own perfection while taking care of you? Or would it be you being perfect by giving your partner such an opportunity to be revealed as a good man or woman? Do you love others so that you yourself can feel the love? Or do you love so that you can give to another? Do you give to another, in love, so that you have the opportunity to give? Or are you selfish for seizing that opportunity, and therefore you give love? These two polarities of love are so interwoven that the answers to these questions can only be found in the feelings of the one you show love to. If your lover is the one who answers these, then your lover becomes one with yourself in quantum entanglement. If your lover is one with you, then of course you do it all for yourself.

This process is similar when considering the physical and spiritual realms.

The lower ego-self is removed by unifying in the spirit. Because the spiritual realm has a higher ego type pertaining to the fact that all are together as one. That oneness won't let anyone be, having absolute control as unity. This unified control also removes any single being from having control. While there is no lower self, the higher ego consciousness still has lower ego attributes. Singularity in the physical realm has an ego of being 'one micro being' apart from the 'unified macro being' of the spiritual realm. These realms, when they are connected, counteract each other's egos as the forms of micro-ego and macro-ego become contradictory. Neither of them can remain an ego in reflection of their own duality.

To overcome the lower ego, you must learn to let go of attachments. To become one with the higher ego, you must adhere to and hold onto many attachments. To overcome the higher ego, the collective must allow someone within the unity to be singly in control of something. This is why we give ourselves up to unify with GOD. We give up what we had, and then GOD gives us something better in return. (Matthew 19:28-30) (Mark 10:29-31)

Consider the quantum entanglement of your perception of yourself and others.

Are you better than others? Yes, you are in some areas. That is ok to believe. You are a much better being. Why? Because you are allowed to be. You may be better than someone else at smiling. Smiling can be better than a stern face at attracting.

You being better than everyone else may just be something for you to know about. If there comes a time when you need to prove that you are better, then it must be something that others need to learn. It is ok to be better or even the best, especially for educational purposes. It is ok to be you.

Though this is true, when comparing yourself within the limits that you and your current reality demand, you may not want to feel like you are better than others. They may request that you don't consider yourself more or better than them. They may be better. You may find that someone else is better at something than you are. In this example, you have the lesser advantage.

We live within dualities of male, female, up, down, lesser, more, etc. It is important that each of us is better at something, even if we are only better at being ourselves. Better and lesser must remain in order for differences to exist.

We then find in quantum entanglement of greater and lesser that we are brought together in equality. Less becomes more. In food, less spicy may become more desirable. Here, you are only more because you are less. You can be more of a student when you are less educated. Our imperfections become our perfections.

Because of the reality of the manifested universe, there is no such thing as being greater or better. The system of unification doesn't allow for anyone to actually be a better being than someone else. You couldn't have a teacher without a student. The teacher makes the student, and vice versa. We all have different circumstances that we are bound to. If you compare with someone else based on circumstances, then you are both equal. Because of different situations, there is no greater or lesser.

Regardless of what happens, we are always perfect in superficial inadequacies. We are an equilibrium that consists of our purpose being stronger than the standard purposelessness that the universe seemingly unfolds. You are bigger than the entire universe. Though you may seem smaller in scale, all things in existence are the same size.

Consider this. When viewed from light-years away, though you would look microscopic, you are larger than the entire universe put together. You easily dwarf Jupiter and the Milky Way, as well as the entire Virgo Supercluster. Put these gargantuan objects behind you. Now place a camera facing the direction of one of these objects. Get a picture while the camera is only inches away from your body. What you will see is that you can block the view of all other things.

You are more than time; yes, you are. You can move a single rock, and through all time and space, your action will affect the atomic alignment of the physical universe forever. On the opposite spectrum of this foresight, time is so great that it has the ability to record everything.

What you'll find is that you are simultaneously better, equal, and less, based on the emanation that you entered into. You can also be something completely different than those three.

These writings are based in a common sense quantum field, with relatable topics and reflective examinations of common things in life. Don't be discouraged if you don't grasp it all. It is ok to be in the infancy phases of comprehension. Because once you cross one infancy phase and excel through into maturity, you then become an infant in another area beyond that. The beginning is the end, and the end is the beginning. (Revelation 1:8. 21:6, 22:13)

Have you chosen to see and understand the simplicity of the complexity of it all? Visualize quantum entanglement from the philosophical recognition that intricacy is all so basic. This can be found while pondering. These little equative examples are part of the cognitive quantum field. Discover where everything merges as one, and you can intellectually observe entanglement.

Divine Pillars – This term means the two supports that GOD gave us for connecting heaven and Earth.

There are two Divine Pillars of the Kingdom of Heaven: spirituality and religion. These divine pillars each have a symbolic gender, and they are to be adamantly quantum entangled.

Spirituality is the Divine Masculine Pillar. Your spirituality is where you cultivate a personal relationship with GOD. Here the LORD works with you as an individual. In spirituality, you learn how to cleanse and become a more righteous person. You acquire self-control and grow beneficial self-regulations. You learn that you are spiritually special and unique. (Romans 7:14, 8:6) (1 Corinthians 2:13-15, 15:44-46) This doesn't mean that women cannot be spiritual. We each have two lobes of our brain, and we each have masculine and feminine aspects. Although spirituality is your divine masculine side, there is also a feminine side to it.

Religion is the Divine Feminine Pillar. This is found in the Bible where the Church is referred to as Jesus' bride. (Ephesians 5:22-33) Religion is like a spiritual womb in many ways. Humanity enters religion to be taught as if by a mother. This doesn't mean that men shouldn't be religious. Although religion is your divine feminine side, there is also a masculine side to it.

We find in the Bible and many other religious texts that men are often divinely called by and given a purpose. These GOD given purposes include plans, procedures, and regulations for religions. GOD can be fully trusted. These religious guidelines are meant to help stabilize humanity through evolution so that they don't become extinct. Spiritual directions from GOD may include laws, dietary information, and priesthood designs. When a man is called by GOD, the LORD gives him information. The man is then to bring the information to the people as a gift. (Roman's 1:11) (1 Corinthians 9:8-12, 14:12) (Ephesians 1:3) When all GOD given religious keys are brought together, the Kingdom of Heaven is revealed.

Do spiritual people and religions need each other?

Religion is designed to provide a home for spiritual people. Religion is the plan for spirituality, and therefore spirituality without religion is like being a wandering starseed. (Jude 1:12-13) Each seed must be planted in order for it to grow.

Look at the positive and negative on a battery or an AC plug. They seek each other until there is a connection, and then they produce light or whatever their current is connected for. Now look at a common disposable battery from the 20th century. Set it on the table for 10 years. The battery will die on its own without ever producing. Each connection needs its other half, yet that other half needs to be the correct current. You cannot hook a nine-volt smoke detector battery in line with a twelve-volt car battery and expect a quality result. The smaller nine-volt would probably burn up.

Then look at all negatives and positives. Spiritual and physical opposites are each looking for their other half. If they connect to their counterpart, they will produce. If they connect to the incorrect current, they lack the ability to produce, or they could burn up. For this reason, GOD chooses specific spiritual people to give them guidance. Spiritual beings and religions both also need their other half.

Many people become spiritual and cast out all religion. Consider the ways that the universe works. We all need each other. Who grows your food? Who ships your food to you? Who provides electricity? Who builds the houses? You could say that we should do it all ourselves. At the rate of doing everything yourself, humanity would go extinct without ever getting off the planet before the sun is gone. That is why GOD gives us direction on how to build a kingdom that will outlast the solar system.

Imagine things that you love, such as the great monuments built by your ancestors. They were built by groups of people working together. Similarly, on an atomic or molecular level, a natural structure such as Mount Everest was built by many elements working together. A single atom couldn't build the entire earth all alone. A single atom, or starseed, is without the purpose of structure. Where would your seed be planted? Religion is needed. Religion provides the ability for manifested direction. If you want to build a very nice spiritual home, you need many people. You will need designers and laborers of many skills. Each individual needs to be spiritual when building a marvelous home. (1 Peter 2:4-8) (Proverbs 9:1-6, 24:3-4)

One of your purposes here is to anchor these feminine and masculine pillars together so that they can unite in cooperation. Your job is to help stop war. Religion without spirituality fights for control. When we anchor the masculine into the feminine and willingly master self-discipline, the control voluntarily flows with ease. That is why it is important for both of these pillars to unite.

Consider the conception and purpose of your existence. The spiritual realm was first created before you were born in the spiritual realm. After the spiritual realm was created, the physical realm came next. You then entered this physical realm as a spiritual servant. Your job here is to connect and merge the spiritual and physical realms. That way you can physically exist as a spiritual being within a spiritual/physical reality.

The spiritual realm is the feminine and, like religion, is all together as one. The physical realm is masculine, and like spirituality while here, it has separate increments. The realms must be connected to complete GODs plan for us.

There are two primary forms of spiritual. Women hold one, and men hold the other. When they come together in quantum entanglement, they create life. On a physical level, this is known as having children through impregnation and birth. Life changes when the child exits the womb.

Throughout history, men and women have often attempted to break away from one another. The separation of men and women caused death in the beginning. To merge them increases life. Like these realms, men and women both fully need each other. Neither one can do this alone. Man needs woman to learn, and vice versa. She is the emotion, and he is the logic. You need them both. You must build up your masculine cognitive knowledge and your emotional intellect. They create an equilibrium. Being together is part of uniting the spiritual and physical realms.

The spiritual realm has eternal life, while the physical realm builds souls and recognizable beings. You can live in the Spirit, yet your life is proposed to exist because of the physical realm. It is a paradox. In quantum entanglement, the spiritual and physical realms come together. This brings life to the physical domain. It also brings experience and types of existence to the spiritual realm.

We all have a big job to do, and each of us must do our part. Some of us have the job of just experiencing so that understanding can be recorded and analyzed. That analytical data is then handed to people who do the work of merging the realms. Everyone should be doing their share.

Why don't religions get along with each other like spiritual people do?

Most religions currently claim that their prophet or founder(s) was/were the final say in the entirety of religious future. Here are some examples. Most Christian denominations, such as Catholicism, claim that there hasn't been any revelation since the Apostle Paul. Jehovah's witnesses teach that all other churches are apostate and that they are the only true one. 7th Day Adventists believe that their first church leaders were called by GOD to found their church and have taught that they were the end of messages from GOD. Mormons teach that Joseph Smith was the final say in religion. Muslims believe that Muhammad was the final messenger. Cao Dai is considered the third and final revelation. Each religion sealed themselves and shut the man out, consequently having shut GOD out. There is a common belief in religions that GOD and angels don't talk to people anymore. They unknowingly shut out future growth and made themselves confused. Many of them denounced and hated one another. (1 Corinthians 14:33)

Religions have the essence of spirituality, yet spirituality has nearly perished within them. Through spiritual enlightenment, people have been given the information to build religions. Though that is true, spirituality isn't the regulations that GOD gives us. Spirituality is the cleansing that we do to become spiritual beings. Spirituality includes obedience to GOD. It is about freely giving to others, such as those in need. Spirituality is about helping the poor. Spirituality is about being honest with yourself and others. It increases the nurturing, the care, the kindness, and the thoughtfulness of everything you are. Spirituality is GOD's personal relationship with each of us. It is needed. When a religion says that no one else will get a message from GOD, they cast out the personal relationship aspect. GOD chooses.

If religion attempted to exist without spirituality, religion would stop evolving. There wouldn't be any change, or righteous purpose, and therefore they wouldn't be able to progress beyond being a controlled group. Religion without spirituality would have a sense of emptiness. They would use regulation and restraint without reason. Self-seeking would become the goal. Each religion would also seek their own group and attempt to leave the other spiritual houses out. (Romans 2:5-11) (James 3:14-16) This would lead to war for dominion over command. Evidence of this happening is found when a religious group claims that one of their leaders is the only access to GOD. We know that GOD can choose anyone to receive revelation. Religions begin dying when they refuse GOD's choice in this. (Daniel 4:17)

Why do religions stop producing new revelations as soon as they are born?

Religious leaders often shut GOD out. One reason for this is that GOD's ways are not always attractive to those in leadership positions. Leaders have often denied messages from GOD so that they can retain their personal authority. They choose earthly ways instead of heavenly ways. (John 3:12) The leaders teach their doctrines as the commandments of earthly ideas. (Matthew 15:9) When leaders use human reason to guide the religions, they often become barren. For instance, if a military officer, such as a marine, guides a church, the spirituality in the church dies. Spirituality leads to ideas such as love, anti-war, inner peace, and veganism. There is no spirituality in using a gun to solve human conflict. Those who believe in the ways of the gun have a different system of thought. When religion goes under the control of worldly governments, they no longer listen to GOD. It isn't always the more attractive path to listen to GOD. Religions are required to completely detach from being guided by governments and officers. That is where most religions fail immediately. The people want to honor those who have served in battle. GOD teaches that if we honor those who battled in war, then the war becomes the seed that they have planted. A war veteran cannot teach people spirituality unless he or she has completely denounced that path.

Who then can an established house trust as their next revelator when so many people claim to be from GOD? The truth is, GOD will send proof if someone has a real message. One form of proof that someone works for GOD is in their detachment from all worldly governments. A second form of proof that someone works for GOD, is that they don't meddle in governmental affairs. They don't do things such as vote in politics or hang national flags of worldly countries. They don't promote military service or work in governmental positions. They adhere to paths of spirituality and religion, and that is what they teach the people.

There are different types of foods. Each doctrine is considered a food. The commandments of men are worldly governmental regulations. We are told not to touch, taste, or handle their doctrines. This includes all of their laws, politics, and wars. (Colossians 2:22) (Titus 1:4)

It is the job of the religious leaders to be watchers. They are to watch for anyone having the next piece of GOD's direction. (Jeremiah 6:17) Each religion is supposed to test every man who claims to have been called by GOD. They are to listen well and give each person declaring to have been called an honest chance to see if their calling is true. The religions were not doing this. Their leaders in charge were quite often the ones that GOD was denying. They usually didn't want anything to do with GOD. They wanted to be in charge of GOD's house, yet didn't want GOD to be in charge of them. They didn't want to reflect in truth.

Quantum Sanctity – This term means holiness within your auric field frequency. In order to gain quantum sanctity, you must cleanse your eight body spaces and be in tune with GOD. It is essential that you are in alignment with the timeline of your greatest path. You need to have planted your starseed into the collective consciousness.

After you are cleansed, you may put your frequency into the cosmos and enter the Kingdom of Heaven. There are many ways to do this. Planting your starseed could be as simple as doing your best to help reforest the world. You can enter the collective consciousness of humanity and anchor your new frequency into a soul family. You may even choose to enter a religion. Only you and GOD know how to plant your seed. Others can only help guide and offer advice.

Body Spaces – This term means the areas of consciousness in which you hold your actions, thoughts, and behavioral patterns.

You have eight primary body spaces that together make up who you are. Each of these eight spaces is a body of information, frequencies, people, places, things, thoughts, actions, etc. You can use your body spaces as a series of navigation systems. Together they are your adamant body space of the Way of Love.

What do you want to embody? Are you personifying the you that you desire to be? Cultivating a connection with your eight body spaces is essential. Your body spaces are like vessels that help you navigate through life. Each of these spaces holds a form of your intelligence. Check your body spaces, making sure that you are doing your best to maintain each of them. Develop healthy connections within all of these. Do the internal work to build them, and the world around you will respond.

Emotional/Heart Body Space – Your emotional body, also known as your heart body, is where you hold your heart space. This is the space where you allow emotions to be felt and where you express and let emotions in. You may hold certain people and ideas within your heart space, while others you may not. You may have rules of what you allow yourself to love. Those rules are part of your heart space. If you find yourself loving a destructive idea, you could remove it from your heart space. Your feminine emotional space is in alignment with knowledge, and your masculine emotional space is in alignment with wisdom.

Physical Body Space – Your physical body is where you hold your physical space. It is the space where you allow physical contact. It is where you allow things to enter your body and where physical actions occur. Your body space may include eating healthy, exercising, and other beneficial habits. Your physical space is in alignment with discretion.

Doctrinal Body Space – Your doctrinal body is where you hold your belief systems. It is the space where you allow beliefs to be integrated together. Your doctrine is your system or body of beliefs. Your doctrinal space is in alignment with instruction.

Spirit Body Space – Your spirit body is where you hold your spiritual connections. It is the place where you allow your spirit to reciprocate, infuse, recalibrate, and transmute with yours. This is the area of your vibrational energetic frequency. This isn't the same as your Spirit, yet it is the space in which you allow interaction with your Spirit. Your Spirit is your divine being and your personality. Your spirit space is in alignment with counsel.

Mental Body Space – Your mental body is where you store thoughts and information that you have learned. It is the place where you allow new data to be gathered. It is where you cognitively think. You can increase your mental space by practicing things such as mathematics. Your feminine mental space is in alignment with wisdom, and your masculine mental space is in alignment with knowledge.

Soul Body Space of Light – Your soul body is where you hold memories of your experiences. It is the place where you allow events to enter your life. Your soul is a recording of your experience during this life and any other lives that you may have lived. Your soul space is closely linked to your social space and remains in alignment with perception inside your psychological atomic nucleus. This atomic alignment signifies memories of experiences being processed and recorded.

Social Body Space of Light – Your social body is where you hold your social connections. It is the place where you allow pets, friends, family, and society to enter your life. Your social and soul bodies are both part of your body of light. Your social space is in alignment with understanding.

Body of Works (Workspace) – Your body of works is your accumulated works throughout life. It is the space where you do things for others and for the greater good of humanity. Your job is held within your body of works. Your workspace is in alignment with equity.

Body Space of the Way of Love – Your body of the Way of Love is in reflection of all your ways put together. It is the space where the way that you love is reflected throughout yourself and the conscious collective of humanity. It holds your entire purpose, mission, and path. It holds the idea of what and who you are. Your way of love is in alignment with prudence.

Circuit of Masculine and Feminine Body Spaces

Masculine and feminine body spaces are different. The feminine body spaces are aligned to the proton heart. The masculine body spaces are aligned to the proton mind. Each of the eight bodies in masculine and feminine are different in both word and life. These two proton types plug into each other to bring word and life together. (John 1:1-5)

In the masculine proton mind, word encompasses most of reality. The masculine mind has life in the heart space of their body of works. In the feminine proton heart, life encompasses most of reality. The feminine heart has word in the heart space of their body of works. These two opposite types of proton genders complement one another. When men and women come together, their word aligns with their life. There is much more information about proton hearts and minds within books 7, 10, and 12 of this series.

Masculine Proton Mind

Emotional Body (Heart Body) (Life)

Physical Body (Word)

Doctrinal Body (Word)

Spirit Body (Word)

Mental Body (Word)

Soul Body (Body of Light) (Word)

Social Body (Body of Light) (Word)

Body of Works (Life)

Feminine Proton Heart

Emotional Body (Heart Body) (Word)

Physical Body (Life)

Doctrinal Body (Life)

Spirit Body (Life)

Mental Body (Life)

Soul Body (Body of Light) (Life)

Social Body (Body of Light) (Life)

Body of Works (Word)

These feminine and masculine body spaces are aligned to the Urim and Thummim of the quantum field. More about the Urim and Thummim can be found in Book 7 of this series.

Cosmic Portals

These are the twelve cosmic portals. Most people had been celebrating these portals based on the months that the standard calendar uses. These portals have been connected to the cosmic vortex through the solstices and equinoxes. They were also aligned to the perihelion and aphelion with the Aurora Calendar. The perihelion and aphelion cycle through time, which allows portal evolution. More about the Aurora calendar can be found in Book 7 of this series.

These cosmic portals are special days to get together and express quality frequencies. Twelve gateways are timed into energetic zones. These are not holidays or required moments to get together. These are not times for doing witchcraft or seances. The idea is that you have twelve days to gather, celebrate, and encourage each other's constructive vibes.

December 22th is the 1:1 Portal.

January 20nd is the 2:2 Portal. (January 21st on leap years)

February 21st is the 3:3 Portal. (February 22nd on leap years)

March 24th is the 4:4 Portal.

April 24th is the 5:5 Portal.

May 26th is the 6:6 Portal.

June 27th is the 7:7 Portal.

July 30th is the 8:8 Portal.

August 31st is the 9:9 Portal.

October 2nd is the 10:10 Portal.

November 2nd is the 11:11 Portal.

December 3rd is the 12:12 Portal.

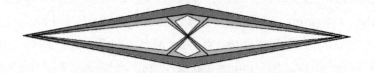

Chapter 3
Divinely Aligned Chakras and Auras

In this chapter you will find the chakra and aura systems scientifically integrated.

When studying the chakras and how they linked to colors and musical notes, it was found that the information varied. There wasn't a definite note for each chakra. In finding a precise unison, the colors were scientifically fused with the correct musical notes. To do this, the frequencies of the notes were increased forty octaves until they precisely aligned with the correct color. The information on how this was done can be found on these two mentioned sites.

https://www.endolith.com/wordpress/2010/09/15/a-mapping-between-musical-notes-and-colors/

https://muted.io/note-frequencies/

The chakras and auras are now accurately merged with the Urim and Thummim. They were then integrated with the correct vibrations and colors so that they are all scientifically consistent. This system is the same alignment used in Book 7 of this series for the entire galactic map. That means that the chakras, auras, astrology, frequencies, and colors are all in scientific and spiritual harmony. The previous systems used were prototypes, which is why they varied. This system is quantum shifted into the new Earth.

This Gnostic quote helps us comprehend why correspondence is needed.

(Gnostic The Tripartite Tractate) "Truth, since it is a unity and multiplicity, receives honor in the small and the great names according to the power of each to grasp it - by way of analogy - like a spring which is what it is, yet flows into streams and lakes and canals and branches, or like a root spread out beneath trees and branches with its fruit, or like a human body, which is partitioned in an indivisible way into members of members, primary members and secondary, great and small."

CODEX I Translated by Harold W. Attridge and Dieter Mueller Selection made from James M. Robinson, ed., The Nag Hammadi Library, revised edition. HarperCollins, San Francisco, 1990.

Alignments in this book are much different than conventionally taught. The reason for this is because wavering information generates inaccuracy. These systems and techniques are precisely aligned with source. Here you can step into the very point of creation and tune into SOURCE FREQUENCY. When you do so, GOD hears your prayers. (Psalm 4:3) The entire system of books 7 and 8 of this series is sealed directly to source. The very point of creation and the tuning can be found in Book 12 of this series.

This guide was designed for spiritual coaching. The information holds the coordinates for your chakras and auras. It is put together in a raw form, keeping it simple and accurate. Even if you are not a professional coach, anyone can use this doctrine.

You have the ability to radiate every aura color. Depending on factors such as your mood or job, your aura can shift periodically. You may also emit multiple colors at the same time.

How do you find your current color? Consider that some people can see auras while others may not. The chakras are the coordinates of your auras. For those who cannot see the colors, these alignments allow us to observe them without the visual eye.

The information for each chakra is calibrated to your aura colors. This way you can find the coordinates of your auric signatures. Lists of focuses and stabilizers are provided so that you can cleanse and strengthen each area. These lists are divinely synchronized.

If someone were having a problem in an area of their life, the coach is able to use the chakra data to see which color resonance their problem aligns to. The coach would then help them correct their difficulties using the focus and stabilizer lists for their auras. These two lists are found in the chakra alignments. In general, the focuses need to be cleansed and strengthened. Each person should recognize, comprehend, participate in, and practice gratitude towards the stabilizers.

When using the frequencies, sometimes the next level of vibration can be applied to help conduct the achievement of the previous chakra guide. (Psalm 61:2)

Cleansing and reinforcing each area of your chakras is important so that you can proceed to the next resonance. When observing a zone that isn't easy to fortify because of missing family connections, you may find the connections within yourself.

Each chakra has a second set of ascension frequencies. When you see those who are in lower resonance, you can help them achieve their goals and elevate their vibration.

1: Lower Infrared/Dark Red – Taproot Earth Star Ma Chakra

This is the first outer ancestral taproot chakra. Here you stand as if on the ground with your sandals. (Exodus 3:5) (Acts 7:33)

This chakra is connected to frequencies between a minute 0.01 Hz and 381 Hz. The primary taproot note is 369.99 Hz F#. Some of the sacred notes eminent in this chakra are 174.61 Hz F solfeggio, 220 Hz A, and 285 Hz solfeggio.

Once ascended, this chakra radiates infrasound and an extremely low frequency (ELF) between 3 Hz and 30 Hz. You will also radiate far infrared (FIR) and mid infrared (MIR) frequencies between 300 GHz and 30 THz while helping your child ascend in growth. These are expressive frequencies that alter the quality of your surrounding reality in good ways.

This chakra emerges with one- to three-petal flowers, including the calla and mariposa lilies. We begin with one to three petals, each signifying a single person.

This is the chakra that you reside in with your mom.

If your mom's frequency is ascended, and she resonates with your dad, your love becomes unbreakable with your parents. This indestructible love is signified by the 220 Hz triangle wave frequency. Triangles are the only shape that do not adjust with pressure, hence the threefold strength of the two parents with their child.

Infrared/Dark Red Taproot Aura

The taproot aura color is infrared through dark red, around 174-0-0.

Here is where you ride your mom's aura.

Your taproot aura is about your dad's mind being in your mom's heart and how it affects you. The feminine side of your being processes and expresses thought with the heart. The masculine side of your being processes and expresses emotion with the mind. This aura is regulated by the way your mom accepts your dad's loving mind. His mind is his heart, and her heart is her mind. Your red aura will be greatly stabilized if you learn through your parents being receptive of one another.

When you become an adult, this aura radiates throughout life, reflecting the way you accept love from the masculine mind. This aura is linked to your fountain of youth.

Celestial Sphere Alignment – Luna
Elemental Alignment – Vocal Power

2: Upper Red – Sinker Root Earth Star Pa Chakra

This is the second outer ancestral sinker root chakra. Here you stand on your feet as yourself while following others. (Jeremiah 30:21)

This chakra is connected to frequencies between 381 Hz and 403 Hz. The primary sinker root note is 392 Hz G. 396 Hz solfeggio is a sacred frequency in this chakra.

Once ascended, this chakra radiates a super low frequency (SLF) between 30 Hz and 300 Hz. This is an expressive frequency that alters the quality of your surrounding reality in good ways.

This chakra emerges with three- and four-petal flowers, including henna blooms known as lawsonia inermis. (Song of Solomon 1:14)

This is the chakra that you reside in with your dad.

If your dad's frequency is ascended, and he resonates with your mom, the two earth star chakras become binary. The earth star chakras then become one earth star. This is how your love becomes unbreakable with your parents. The indestructible love is signified by the mom, dad, and child connecting in the 220 Hz triangle wave frequency of the earth star ma chakra.

You will also radiate mid infrared (MIR) and near infrared (NIR) frequencies between 30 THz and 480 THz while helping your child ascend in growth. These are expressive frequencies that alter the quality of your surrounding reality in good ways.

Red Sinker Root Aura

Here is where you ride your dad's aura.

The sinker root aura color is infrared through red around 255-0-0. This is the same color as the base aura. Because of this, the dad is the mom's access point to being able to guide the future of the life of the child. When the mom resonates with the dad, she can guide the child's path.

Your sinker root aura is about your mom's heart being in your dad's mind and how it affects you. The feminine side of your being processes and expresses thought with the heart. The masculine side of your being processes and expresses emotion with the mind. This aura is regulated by the way your dad accepts your mom's loving heart. His mind is his heart, and her heart is her mind. Your red sinker root aura will be greatly stabilized if you learn through your parents being receptive of one another.

When you become an adult, this aura radiates through life, reflecting the way you accept love from the feminine heart. This aura is linked to your fountain of youth.

Red Sinker Root Aura Focus

The sinker root aura color is dark red, around 174-0-0, and red, around 255-0-0.
1: Motivation.
2: Promoting the common good.

This aura can be affected by who your dad was and how his resonation aligned with your mom before you were conceived. Your lower earth star aura can be affected by who your mom was and how her resonation aligned with your dad's before you were conceived. Your parents may not seem to express a loving resonance. Some people don't even know their parents. If you feel that you have a disconnection in this area, you can still find them loving one another. Their binary earth star lives within you.

Celestial Sphere Alignment – Helios
Elemental Alignment – Voice

3: Red Lateral Root Base Chakra

This is the lateral root base chakra of wisdom. It is the fundamental negative or psychological electron. It emphasizes survival. This chakra includes spiritual connectedness of the body and our personal needs. It is a flowing brook of life and your connection to the Holy Ghost and divine feminine.

The masculine side of the Lateral Root Chakra is the primary emotional wisdom.

The feminine side of the Lateral Root Chakra is the primary cognitive wisdom.

This chakra is connected to frequencies between 403 Hz and 427 Hz. The primary lateral root note is 415.3 Hz G#. 417 Hz solfeggio is a sacred frequency in this chakra.

Once you have ascended, this chakra radiates an ultra low frequency (ULF) between 300 Hz and 3 kHz. This is an expressive frequency that alters the quality of your surrounding reality in good ways. When your lateral root chakra is ascended, it emphasizes the survival and needs of others.

This chakra emerges with four- and five-petal flowers, including the rose of Sharon. (Song of Solomon 2:1)

Red Lateral Root Aura Focus

The lateral root aura color is red, around 255-0-0.

1: Planning and preparation.

2: Equal opportunities and compassion.

3: Self-reflection.

4: Reflective perspectives.

5: Becoming a living success in helpful ways.

6: Taking care of our hearts so we (and others) can have a great journey.

7: Being genuine and loving your life for what it is.

This aura can be affected by who your mom was and how she resonated with your dad before you were conceived.

Red Lateral Root Aura Stabilizers

Construction and building that men do.

Construction and building that women do.

Celestial Sphere Alignments – Venus and Neptune

Elemental Alignment – Metal

4: Orange Bole/Trunk Sacral Chakra

This is the bole/trunk sacral chakra of discretion. It is the fundamental mass and/or volume. It emphasizes the relationship between electron and proton. This chakra includes spiritual connectedness of the body. It is a flowing brook of life and your connection to the Holy Spirit, divine union of masculine and feminine.

The trunk chakra is where the masculine and feminine meet in the emotional cognitive discretion.

This chakra is connected to frequencies between 427 Hz and 453 Hz. The primary trunk note is 440 Hz G#. 432 Hz is a sacred frequency in this chakra.

Once you have ascended, this chakra radiates a very low frequency (VLF) between 3 kHz and 30 kHz. This is an expressive frequency that alters the quality of your surrounding reality in good ways.

This chakra emerges with five- to seven-petal flowers, including lily, lily of the valleys, and the hyacinthus. (Song of Solomon 2:1)

Orange Trunk Aura Focus

The trunk aura color is orange, around 255-102-0.

1: Routine decisions.

2: Personal decisions.

3: Strategic decisions.

4: Organizational decisions.

5: Being full of positive, loving opinions.

6: Keeping the heart of your mentality in an eventful direction.

This aura can be affected by how your parents treat one another.

Orange Trunk Aura Stabilizer

Final decisions in life.

Celestial Spheres – Ceres and Makemake

Elemental Alignment – Earth

5: Yellow Limb Solar Plexus Chakra

This is the limb chakra of the navel, the solar plexus, and instruction. It is the fundamental divisive transfer. It emphasizes the heartbeat. It is the river of life and your connection to the Spirit and divine masculine.

The masculine side of the limb chakra is the primary cognitive instruction.

The feminine side of the limb chakra is the primary emotional instruction.

This chakra is connected to frequencies between 453 Hz and 480 Hz. The primary limb note is 466.16 Hz A#.

Once you have ascended, this chakra radiates a low frequency (LF) between 30 kHz and 300 kHz. This is an expressive frequency that alters the quality of your surrounding reality in good ways. Here is where we listen to the sacred notes of others.

This chakra emerges with seven- to ten-petal flowers.

Yellow Limb Aura Focus

The limb aura color is yellow, around 255-239-0.

1: Observing and asking questions.

2: Being obedient and submissive to good will.

3: Making correct choices.

4: Being artistic and innovative.

5: Being direct and forthright with kindness.

6: Being friendly and patient-minded.

7: Seeking helpful types of education and paying attention to others.

8: Being protective of others.

9: Being careful and mindful of your surroundings.

10: Paying close attention to others and learning.

11: Formal education.

12: Non-formal education.

13: Sharing with others.

14: Community and assembly. Doing great things with others.

15: Setting aside a moment to do something special for someone.

16: Sharing resources, both spiritual and physical, to help others up in life.

17: Equilibrium of sharing what we can and must, both spiritually and physically.

This aura can be affected by the instructions that your parents gave you.

Yellow Limb Aura Stabilizers

Major decisions that women make.

Resources and helping those in need.

Celestial Sphere Alignments – Vesta and Pluto

Elemental Alignment – Air (Wind)

6: Green Branch True Heart Chakra

This is the branch chakra of the true heart and of knowledge. It is the fundamental positive or psychological proton. It is the breath of life and your connection to the Spirit and divine masculine.

The masculine side of the branch chakra is the primary cognitive knowledge.

The feminine side of the branch chakra is the primary emotional knowledge.

This chakra is connected to frequencies between 508 Hz and 538 Hz. The primary branch note is 523.25 Hz C. 528 Hz solfeggio is a sacred frequency in this chakra.

Once you have ascended, this chakra radiates a high frequency (HF) between 3 MHz and 30 MHz. This is an expressive frequency that alters the quality of your surrounding reality in good ways.

This chakra emerges with ten- to twelve-petal flowers.

Green Branch Aura Focus

The branch aura color is green, around 40-255-0.
(These focuses are precisely linked to the white and chartreuse auras.)
1: Declarative knowledge.
2: Priori and a posteriori – clear reason.
3: Para Vidya (House of the knowledge of GOD).
4: Apara Vidya (founding knowledge of intellect and worldwide advancements).
5: Advancing spiritually and technologically in helpful ways.
6: Resourcefulness and the ability to enjoy life with what we have.

This aura can be affected by how your dad reacted to your birth.

Green Branch Aura Stabilizer

Men gathering information by listening to those in need.

Celestial Sphere Alignments – Eris and Mars
Elemental Alignment – Oxygen

7: Cyan Twig Throat Chakra

This is the twig chakra of the throat and of perception. It is the fundamental pressure connecting the proton and neutron within the psychological atomic nucleolus. This chakra includes spiritual connectedness of the soul and social life. It is the water of life and your connection to the Spirit and divine masculine.

The masculine side of the twig chakra is the primary social emotional perception.

The feminine side of the twig chakra is the primary social cognitive perception.

This chakra is connected to frequencies between a 538 Hz and 570 Hz. The primary twig note is 554.37 Hz C#. 544.4 Hz and 545.6 Hz are sacred frequencies in this chakra.

Once you have ascended, this chakra radiates a very high frequency (VHF) between 30 MHz and 300 MHz. This is an expressive frequency that alters the quality of your surrounding reality in good ways.

This chakra emerges with twelve- to sixteen-petal flowers.

Cyan Twig Aura Focus

The twig aura color is cyan, around 0-255-242.

1: Finding your place in this world; your position in life.
2: Recognition of others.
3: Healthy stimulations.
4: Good memories and how they affect you.
5: Bringing thoughtful life dreams into reality for everyone.
6: Holding people together socially in a positive way.

This aura can be affected by how your dad keeps the family together as one.

Cyan Twig Aura Stabilizer

Women gathering information by listening to those in need.

Celestial Sphere Alignments – Haumea and Mercury
Elemental Alignment – Water

8: Blue Leaf Third Eye Chakra

This is the brow foliage/leaf chakra of the third eye and understanding. It is the fundamental multiplicative and psychological neutron. This chakra includes spiritual connectedness of the soul and social life. It is the wellspring of life and your connection to the Holy Spirit, divine union of masculine and feminine.

The masculine side of the twig chakra is the primary social emotional understanding.

The feminine side of the twig chakra is the primary social cognitive understanding.

This chakra is connected to frequencies between 570 Hz and 640 Hz. The primary twig notes are 587.33 Hz D and 622.25 Hz D#. 639 Hz solfeggio is a sacred frequency in this chakra.

Once you have ascended, this chakra radiates an ultra high frequency (UHF) between 300 MHz and 3 GHz. This is an expressive frequency that alters the quality of your surrounding reality in good ways.

This chakra emerges with 16- to 95-petal flowers.

Blue Twig Aura Focus

The twig aura colors are light blue, around 0-122-255, and dark blue, around 5-0-255.

1: Coworkers (classmates, teammates, etc.) (Dark Blue Aura).

2: Friends – Being Grounded (Light Blue Aura).

3: Being considerate and helpful.

4: Being open-minded and direct.

5: The spectrum of love.

6: Being honest and loving.

7: Keeping family close.

8: Dedication to family.

9: Confidence in happiness and being consistent.

10: Bringing people together.

11: Active listening (Light Blue Aura).

12: Effective communication (Dark Blue Aura).

13: Keeping relationships together.

14: Bringing relationships together to reflect on.

15: Social abilities of bonding beyond your immediate family.

16: Protecting everyone in fair ways.

17: How your social groups can affect you for the better.

This aura can be affected by how your dad reacted to your birth. It can also be affected by what you learned from your parents and how your social life was with them as a child and growing up.

Blue Aura Stabilizers

Architecture of all kinds that men design.

Architecture of all kinds that women design.

Celestial Sphere Alignments – Pallas Athena and Chiron

Elemental Alignment – Fire

9: Purple Top Crown Chakra – Aurora Borealis

This is the top chakra of the crown of equity. It is the fundamental gravity. This chakra includes spiritual connectedness of the body and the soul and social life. It is the crown of life and your connection to the Holy Ghost and divine feminine.

The masculine side of the crown chakra is the primary social emotional equity.

The feminine side of the crown chakra is the primary social cognitive equity.

This chakra is connected to frequencies between 640 Hz and 718 Hz. The primary crown notes are 659.25 Hz E and 698.46 Hz F. 639 Hz solfeggio is a sacred frequency in this chakra.

Once you have ascended, this chakra radiates a super high frequency (SHF) between 3 GHz and 30 GHz. You will also radiate near ultraviolet (NUV) frequencies between 480 THz and 3 PHz. These are expressive frequencies that alter the quality of your surrounding reality in good ways.

This chakra emerges with 96- to 1,000-petal flowers, including the flower of life. (Song of Solomon 8:12)

Purple Crown Aura Focus

The crown aura colors are light purple, around 71-0-237, and dark purple, around 99-0-178.
1: Self-worth.
2: Equilibrium of kindness.
3: Equality (Light Purple Aura).
4: Good karma (Dark Purple Aura) (This focus is precisely linked to the yellow, white, and chartreuse auras.).
5: Bringing people together in caring ways.
6: Leading in good ways.
7: Being in the world with those we love.

This aura can be affected by how your mom brings the family together as one.

Purple Crown Aura Stabilizer

Major decisions that men make.

Celestial Sphere Alignments – Juno and Saturn
Elemental Alignment – Cloud

10: White Ultraviolet 1ˢᵗ Physical Trigon – Soul Star Halo Chakra

This is the center soul star halo chakra of the 1ˢᵗ trigon of prudence. It is the fundamental cognitive weight. It emphasizes your connection between heaven and Earth and selflessness by placing others first. It is the well of life and your connection to the Holy Spirit, divine union of masculine and feminine.

This halo chakra is where the masculine and feminine unite in social prudence.

This chakra is connected to frequencies between 718 Hz and 951 Hz. The primary halo notes are 739.99 Hz F#, 783.99 Hz G, 880 Hz A, and 932.33 Hz A#. Solfeggio notes 741 Hz and 852 Hz are sacred frequencies in this chakra.

Once you have ascended, this chakra radiates an extremely high frequency (EHF) between 30 GHz and 3 THz. You will also radiate extreme ultraviolet (EUV) frequencies between 30 PHz and 3 EHz for ascension. These are expressive frequencies that alter the quality of your surrounding reality in good ways.

This chakra emerges with 1,000- to 10,000-petal flowers.

Ultraviolet/Dark Red Halo Aura Focus

The crown aura color is ultraviolet and dark red, around 174-0-0.
(These focuses are precisely linked to the Earth star auras and the other two ultraviolet trigons.)
1: Common knowledge (common wisdom and understanding).
2: Self-transcendence.
3: Artistic abilities; music, art, etc.
4: Loving your life for everything it is.

This aura can be affected by what you know and how you feel about your parents and how they were emotionally, cognitively, and socially interactive with you.

Ultraviolet/Dark Red Halo Aura Stabilizer

Technological design of all kinds that women design.

Celestial Sphere Alignment – Uranus
Elemental Alignment – Adamant

11: White Ultraviolet 2nd Spiritual Trigon – Spirit Halo Chakra

This is the center spirit halo chakra of the 2nd trigon of prudence. It is the fundamental emotional weight. It emphasizes your connection between heaven and Earth and selflessness by placing others first. It is the fruit of life and your connection to the Holy Spirit, divine union of masculine and feminine.

This halo chakra is where the masculine and feminine unite cognitive prudence.

This chakra is connected to frequencies between 951 Hz and 1070 Hz. The primary halo notes are 987.77 Hz B and 1046.5 Hz C. 963 Hz is a sacred frequency in this chakra.

Once you have ascended, this chakra radiates x-ray frequencies between 3 THz and 30 THz. You will also radiate soft x-ray (SX) and hard x-ray (HX) frequencies between 30 PHz and 30 EHz for ascension. These are expressive frequencies that alter the quality of your surrounding reality in good ways.

This chakra emerges with 10,000- to 1,000,000-petal flowers.

12: White Ultraviolet 3rd Divine Trigon– Universal Halo Chakra

This is the center universal halo chakra of the 3rd trigon of prudence. It is the fundamental social weight. It emphasizes your connection between heaven and Earth and selflessness by placing others first. It is the way of life and your connection to the Holy Spirit, divine union of masculine and feminine.

This halo chakra is where the masculine and feminine unite emotional prudence.

This chakra is connected to frequencies between 1070 Hz and 30,000 Hz. The primary universal notes are 1174.66 Hz D and found beyond that to 30,000 Hz. 1074 Hz, 1152 Hz, and 2172 Hz are sacred frequencies in this chakra.

Once you have ascended, this chakra radiates gamma-ray frequencies around 30 EHz or more for ascension. This is an expressive frequency that alters the quality of your surrounding reality in good ways.

This chakra emerges with 1,000,000- to 100,000,000-petal flowers.

13: Chartreuse Galactic Stem Chakra – Aurora Australis

This is the galactic stem chakra. It is the fundamental density. It emphasizes helping others. This chakra includes spiritual connectedness through focal fusion. It is the tree of life and your connection to the Holy Spirit, divine union of masculine and feminine.

This chakra is about educating others on the path. While in the galactic chakra, we meet people in the lower heart area between the yellow solar plexus chakra and the green heart chakra. We educate in that area to bring them into the true heart. If they accept their growth, they will continue onward to the upper heart area between the green heart chakra and the cyan throat chakra.

The masculine side of the galactic chakra is the primary emotional counsel.

The feminine side of the galactic chakra is the primary cognitive counsel.

This chakra is connected to frequencies between 480 Hz and 508 Hz. The primary crown note is the 493.88 Hz B. 528 Hz solfeggio is a sacred frequency in this chakra.

Once you have ascended, this chakra radiates a medium frequency (MF) between 300 kHz and 3 MHz. This is an expressive frequency that alters the quality of your surrounding reality in good ways.

This chakra emerges with single petal flowers, including the calla lily, along with a mixture of all flowers.

Once you have ascended, this chakra radiates cosmic ray frequencies from 30,000 Hz to Planck frequency and beyond. This means that we have opened the divine gateway of ascension in the spirit. Our vibrations become connected to the frequencies of GOD. These frequences alter the quality of your surrounding reality in good ways.

Chartreuse Stem Aura Focus

The stem aura color is chartreuse around 153-255-0.

1: Gathering metaknowledge from others.
2: Implicit knowledge.
3: Tacit knowledge of culture – nature and GOD's artistic creations (even spiritual).
4: Explicit knowledge.
5: Educating people about sustaining morals.
6: Educating people about sustaining great ideas.

This aura can be affected by what you learned from your parents about how the world works. Counsel can be given one way and received another way. Yet if your parents Earth star chakras are aligned well, then your learning ability can be effectively increased. If you cannot find your parents earth star chakras aligned in them, you can find it within you.

Chartreuse Stem Aura Stabilizer

Technological design of all kinds that men design.

Chartreuse Connections for Enlightening Auras through Spiritually Educating.

Instructive Connections

(These two focuses are part of the yellow aura focus. They are used to enter the yellow aura of someone else.)

1: Discussion
2: Collaboration

You can strengthen the yellow aura by instructing on ways to interact and learn well together during pregnancy.

Knowledgeable Connection

(This focus is precisely linked to the Earth star auras and the three ultraviolet trigons. It is used to draw people into their green aura and help propel them beyond.)

Self-transcendence

Celestial Sphere Alignments – Gaia and Jupiter
Elemental Alignment – Wood

Divine Gateway

To open the divine gateway, you must do something important for another. You must selflessly help someone in an attempt to permanently better their life.

You must do what you can to plant our portion of trees and rehabilitate the earth. You must do what you can to recycle and remain efficient, thus protecting the health of the earth and everyone.

Those who are in the divine gateway chakra have been recorded in heaven.

The divine gateway chakra radiates 30,000 Hz to Planck frequency and beyond, and in the frequency of the perfect sphere. Since there isn't a frequency to represent this gateway, which we can generally hear, we can use 220 Hz.

Once here, our social life may not bond the same with others anymore, and that alone can wedge into us and attempt to dislodge our path. All chakras are centered in the heart. Because of this, when we detach from forms of immorality, many people may no longer connect with us the same. Love can seem to be stressed upon or taken away. Yet love when true remains. Those detachments are detachments from types of love that were not true to you. Those types of connections are often based on honoring someone's path regardless of it being moral or not. Ascended beings relate to and honor moral paths. If someone cannot connect to you anymore, they may push upon your ways in an attempt to get you to reenter their path. It is important not to allow them to take your success away, or you cannot lead them to success.

This chakra emerges with 100,000,000-petal flowers and beyond.

Celestial Sphere Alignment – Firmament
Elemental Alignment – Sanctity

Chakra Bow

The chakra bow graph reveals the white bow. White occurs when all colors reflect together at once. This graph depicts how we can string the bow, place ourselves as an arrow, pull back, and shoot by ascending to heaven. We begin in red and ascend around counterclockwise through the colors while skipping chartreuse. Orange and cyan are where the bowstring is tied. The arrow is placed in purple and pulled back towards the chartreuse area between green and yellow. While drawing the bow back, we enter the center white chakra. Once we find our center, we then pull back into the chartreuse area, which is where we express the ability and right to educate others. Once we are done counseling in chartreuse, the divine gateway opens, and we shoot, ascending to heaven. In heaven we see that the divine gateway is centered like the white chakra.

As we know, a white light is composed of seven lights abbreviated as VIBGYOR, yet here they are arranged as ROYGBIV to align with the rainbow. This is why the white trigon light is in the center of the seven other sections of color.

The chakra bow can be seen in the graph on the next page.

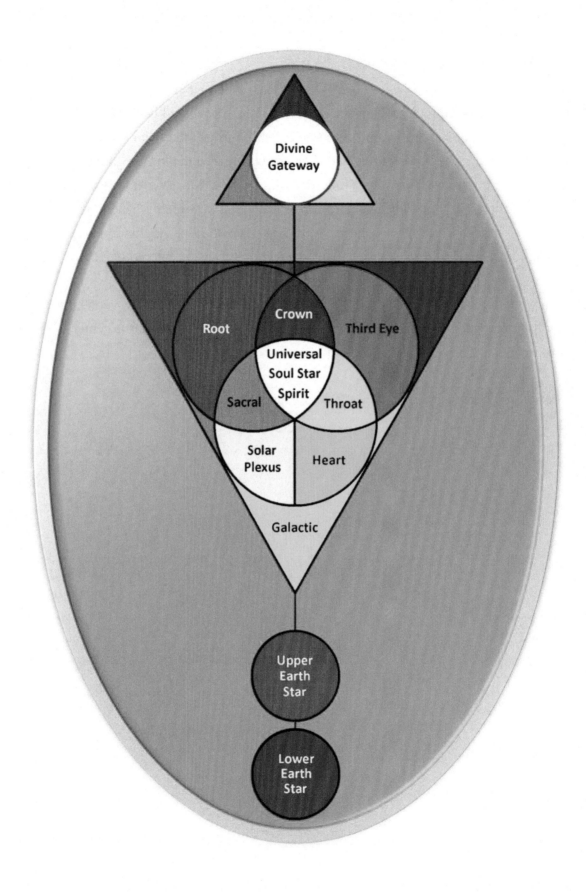

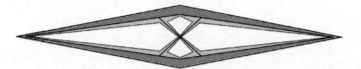

Chapter 4
Sculptor's Diet (Livet)

The ancient Kesh Temple was an ascension sanctuary. This temple had rooms at different levels. Each room signified a chakra. The student would enter a level and learn the frequency there. When the student graduated, they would ascend into the next room above.

The first major form of writing, known as cuneiform, was formed about 3500 BC. This was about 5,500 years ago. The Kesh Temple Hymn was inscribed in cuneiform. The creation of this written language reveals the beginning of an epoch which determined the time to return the Tree of Life.

(Book of Adam and Eve) "O Adam, as to the fruit of the Tree of Life, for which thou askest, I will not give it thee now, but when the 5500 years are fulfilled. Then will I give thee of the fruit of the Tree of Life, and thou shalt eat, and live for ever, thou, and Eve, and thy righteous seed."

It has been said that Adam and Eve were here around 4,000 BC. If that is true, then cuneiform became important when Adam was around 500 years of age. This alignment indicates that it has been about 5,500 years since Adam and Eve began writing history. It is time to return the Tree of Life.

Chapter 25 in Book 7 of this series has a set of questions in Virgo. One question is about who has ascended or descended to return Jesus to the living world. (Romans 10:6-7) It explains that the process of ascension includes a specific diet to be eaten. This book has that diet to share with everyone.

The foods you eat are part of the direct image of the person that you are and the chakra that you are manifested into. Your frequency radiates a reflection of your behavioral pattern. In this chapter, you will find the process of cleansing your body through a divinely tuned diet. Each chakra has a type of food that must be removed when cleansing yourself to the next level.

This chapter has the original proposed nutritional side of the Kesh ascension process. With this diet, along with the quantum field and chakra teachings, you can learn and coach the ascension courses. The Kesh temple plan wasn't ever completed during its day, due to lack of information. Technology needed to complete the temple steps is finally emerging.

Energetic Reiki Cleansing

Everything in the universe has an energetic signature. When you tap a tuning fork against a table, it begins to ring. That ring is a recording of what has happened and is happening to the tuning fork. If you touch the vibrating fork against your arm, the vibration enters you. This is a simple explanation of how energies transfer between people and things.

There are many forms of energetic transfers. You can smile at someone or say something nice to them. It not only makes them happy; their happiness will also radiate back into you. Every time you perform an act of kindness, it helps your health. Everything you do vibrates and reverberates through the universe.

If you come in contact with hatred, you will feel it within you. Hatred can make you sick. Similarly, killing animals generates an energetic expression that enters your body. Each kill is detrimental to your frequency.

Some people use energies for healing purposes. There are various forms of vibrational therapy, including sound healing and Reiki.

Reiki includes sharing the energetic signatures known as auras. When a Reiki practitioner performs a healing session, they share their frequency. To do a successful Reiki session, the practitioner should have very cleansed energy. The patient purposely opens full access to their auric field by trusting and allowing the practitioner to penetrate their frequency. Where the patient and the Reiki professional are agreed as one, their energies merge.

Many Reiki experts operate as a conduit for Source Frequency. (Matthew 18:20) They become a channel between Source and the patient.

Imagine the conduit (practitioner) as a water pipe and Source frequency as the water. If the water pipe is dirty, the water coming through will collect debris. These debris will enter the patient. It is imperative that the practitioner has a cleansed energy.

Reiki therapists can spend time researching and practicing in the spiritual quantum field. They can meditate to remain clean. They may also spend time alone before a session in order to remove external vibrations and unwanted contaminants.

The nutritional path revealed in chapters 4, 5, and 6 of this book was designed to help the practitioner become a clean conduit. This diet, also known as the Livet, has various steps. The Livet assists professionals in connecting to Source energy. It is important that the expert is on an equal or greater dietary level than the patient. Qualified hands in practice should be as clean or cleaner than the patient.

In reflection, the Reiki therapist may intake some of the patient's energy while cleansing their auric field. Know that this can temporarily lower their vibrational health. For this reason, patients should be courteous by cleansing themselves the best they can for the practitioner.

Nutritional Refinement

Lower Infrared/Dark Red – Taproot Earth Star Ma Chakra

Those nutritionally tuned to the lower earth star chakra only eat what the parents feed them. Often this is breast milk. As we grow, we see that we are all here together.

Upper Red – Sinker Root Earth Star Pa Chakra

Those nutritionally tuned to the upper earth star chakra only eat what they are taught to eat by parents and/or other people that the parents allow. This chakra signifies yourself as a child while venturing out under your parents' discretion.

To accomplish the nutritional tuning of the upper earth star chakra, one must be in charge of their own food intake. Then they can move on to cleansing their root base.

Red Lateral Root Base Chakra

Those nutritionally tuned to the root base chakra practice standard diets, which are for survival. These people will eat anything to survive and are at the base or root of existence, often living in the moment.

To accomplish the nutritional tuning of the lateral root chakra, one must become willing to protect themselves and cleanse their base. They must be willing to shield their well-being by eating healthier food. Then they can move on to cleansing their sacral.

Orange Bole/Trunk Sacral Chakra

Those nutritionally tuned to the sacral chakra practice health food diets such as Mediterranean and keto. They generally exclude fast food. These people have chosen to take care of themselves and look to the future instead of just living in the moment.

To accomplish the nutritional tuning of the trunk sacral chakra, one must become willing to protect the futures of others. Then they can move on to cleansing their solar plexus.

Yellow Limb Solar Plexus Chakra

Those nutritionally tuned to the solar plexus chakra practice a pescatarian diet. These people are in range of the lower heart chakra. They choose to apply a higher self-worth and may exude compassion. This compassion is reflected in the fact that they only eat fish, believing that fish don't have feelings nor feel pain. They may believe that fish are not tortured like other animals.

As for eating fish, there was a 1990s song called 'Something In The Way' by a band called Nirvana. In the lyrics it said, "It's OK to eat fish 'cause they don't have any feelings."

Fish are caught in gill nets and with hooks. They are pulled out of the water and slowly suffocated. That would be torture. Watch these four short videos if you would like to know more about the intelligence of fish. Consider these things.

https://youtu.be/vVnE9o5Uxik

https://youtu.be/6at5gBa4ZbI

https://youtu.be/15Xi-IUKj7A

https://youtu.be/1k0MMxhOVpA

You may notice that the primary limb note is 466.16 Hz A#. The oldest known version of the part of the biblical book of Revelation which speaks of the number of the beast says 616 instead of 666. This is found in papyrus 115. What this note means when scientifically aligned in the chakras is that those eating meat, including fish, are still participating in beast nature of the animal kingdom.

To accomplish the nutritional tuning of the limb solar plexus chakra, one must become willing to care for other sentient beings. Then they can move on to cleansing their true heart.

Green Branch True Heart Chakra

Those nutritionally tuned to the true heart chakra practice a vegetarian diet. Their energy and personality have entered the true heart, and they no longer want to kill conscious beings. They stop eating fish and want to be kind. One cannot nutritionally tune this chakra while killing animals, because the killing is a direct reflection of their energetic path. Whatever your vibrational energy is, it precisely reproduces, reveals, and exposes your chakra's frequency into your manifested reality.

According to the ancient rules from the LORD, vegetarianism is the legally acceptable minimum for nutritional guidelines. This guideline is based on your animals being your friends. There is a difference between a friend sharing some milk and just caging animals and robbing them. This is better explained in books 6 and 12 of this series.

To accomplish the nutritional tuning of the true heart chakra, one must choose not to steal from others, including all sentient beings, and cleanse their heart. Then they can move on to cleansing their throat.

Cyan Twig Throat Chakra

Those nutritionally tuned to the throat chakra practice veganism. They progress towards a correct moral revealed by not stealing from animals. Vegans no longer take from babies. They let their mothers feed them. And the little bees are safe to play in the flowers while filling their honeybanks. Bees work hard for their food and provide much for everyone by pollinating. Insects and animals are babies and children when compared to human intelligence. Vegans learn not to take advantage of them. Vegans no longer eat dairy, honey, or other animal products and avoid using them. Vegans have safe passage.

Through personal observation of claims, the author of this book hasn't ever seen anyone's third eye opened unless they were vegan. Though they claim that they do, they seem to not know what it means.

Vegans find that since they don't take from others, they need to supplement with vitamins D-3, K-2, and B-12. They use their elevated intelligence to provide these micronutrients.

What vegans speak can overcome. Their voices can be clean.

Those who are vegan may easily comprehend the difference between their throats and the throats of meat eaters as in these verses. (Psalm 5:9) (Romans 3:13)

To accomplish the nutritional tuning of the throat chakra, one must place that which is healthy before that which feels or tastes best.

Blue Leaf Third Eye Chakra

Those nutritionally tuned to the third eye chakra practice diets such as raw veganism and fruitarianism. They exclude fast food. These people can set themselves beyond flavor and open their mind's eye to receive further instruction from the divine.

The best way to open your third eye is by learning to take care of yourself and others at the same time. Another important factor is learning not to allow the five senses to rule your direction.

It does so much for everyone when you become vegan. The health of the entire world is increased by the production of plant-based foods instead of animal products. If you have helped everyone by becoming vegan, you may then also want to do something for yourself. You are a creation from the Divine. Loving yourself is also to love the Divine who created you. When we truly love others and also love ourselves, the Divine opens to us.

The five senses can be a blessing, yet they can also hold us down if the mind isn't in charge of them. The five senses can rule the standard vegan diet of the throat chakra. Once vegans give up meats and dairy products, they often go in search of flavorful foods. Many vegan foods are also processed with chemicals. Raw vegans allow logic and instruction from the Divine to rule over the five senses instead of the other way around.

Those who have their third eye open avoid artificially flavored or chemically altered foods, as well as those with preservatives. They exclude manufactured foods. They exclude bleached foods such as white flour. They eat the best vegan foods that they can instead of going for the most flavor. The third eye isn't necessarily about whether food is cooked or not; rather, the best nutrient value is sought instead of best flavors.

To accomplish the nutritional tuning of the third eye chakra, one must clean the mind of all intoxicants and learn to do their best not to kill plants. Then they can move on to cleansing their crown.

Purple Top Crown Chakra – Aurora Borealis

True love deserves a royal crown of life to align into the OM of nutritional Omnism. There you can honestly love the Divine. (Psalm 103:4) (James 1:12) (Revelation 2:10)

Those in the third eye chakra have done so much for others and have overcome the weaknesses of the 5 senses well. Those who get this far know that they are near doing the best that they can. Those nutritionally tuned to the crown chakra choose not to kill plants for food. In wearing a crown, one must unite the self and the selfless as one. First, we focus on the selfless side of the crown.

To put the crown on a raw vegan or those in such diets, one must not kill plants for food. To do this, you are only to eat what passes of itself. We can avoid eating tubers and roots of any kind, because taking roots kills plants. Eat the greens and/or tops of the plants that grow back again and again without harming the roots. Eat the fruits and vegetables, yet don't kill the plant. Be careful with foods from the sea to protect the coral reefs and keep pollutants out. Palm fruit is also avoided unless very safely sourced. Crown wearers also do what they can not to kill insects.

Next, we will focus on the self-side of the crown. Wearing a crown also means that we stop harming ourselves. While looking into themselves through the third eye chakra, many people often still use intoxicants. Intoxicants such as alcohol, coffee (caffeine), tobacco, stimulants, and medications, both over the counter and prescription (except for in cases of medical emergencies), are avoided by those in the crown chakra.

Once you put the crown chakra on, you are no longer human. You then become an Anno Human. You have evolved into a new species. Your energy frequency and thought process are changed. (Job 14:14)

Those wearing a crown still have safe passage with vitamins D-2, Lichen D-3, K-2, and B-12 based on all chakras aligning correctly. If they have a crown, they are allowed to use bacteria as a mechanism for producing vitamins instead of a plant or animal. With this logic, they can have the vitamins in order to survive. If they were not allowed the bacterial help, then even walking would be problematic because we wouldn't want to harm the bacteria. We must survive so that we can help lead others. Everyone we support saves lives. If we were to lay our root chakra down and die without those vitamins, the truth could die with us. Then there would be no point to life in the first place.

All seven personal chakras must be aligned together and functioning properly to nutritionally cleanse your crown. Those with a nutritionally cleansed crown chakra no longer eat any diet; rather, they eat the Sculptors Livet. This is a crown of Life. (James 1:12)

To accomplish the nutritional tuning of the crown chakra, you must divinely align the crown.

White Ultraviolet 1ˢᵗ Trigon of Rights to Light – Soul Star Halo Chakra

Those nutritionally tuned to the soul star halo chakra practice the Sculptor's Livet. If you have your crown, then you have accomplished the nutritional tuning of the primary seven chakras.

When the chakras are all brought together, they become one. According to the color additive system, all colors together produce white. You can graduate into the soul star chakra where the Livet and nutrition are changed and tuned through divine guidance. In this, they become true, authentic, and sincere to the Divine. Then they can resonate beyond the crown.

Those in the soul star chakra practice a nutritious form of veganism. They exclude pungent vegetables such as onions, green onions, garlic, ginger, chives, and leeks. They exclude cane sugar. They exclude foods that are excessively spicy, sweet, bitter, salty, and sour. They exclude iodized salt and vinegar. They exclude chocolate and bananas. They exclude pomegranates, figs, apples, lumia pear lemons, grapefruits, quinces, poppies, yeast, psychedelic mushrooms, and fungi (other than for extracted supplemental purposes of D-2 and/or D-3). They exclude canned foods unless they are self-canned seeds without preservatives. They exclude wheat (gluten), grapes, melons, cucumbers, and leeks. They exclude fava beans. They also exclude thistles and food from plants that have thorns. Thorns are as if the plant is telling us that it is not for us.

Only natural forms of salt, such as Himalayan and sea salts, are ingested. Sodium is ingested as a supplement based on the measured amount you need daily. Because of this, they will need to supplement with a naturally sourced iodine.

To accomplish the nutritional tuning of the soul star chakra, one must learn to hear the needs of the self.

White Ultraviolet 2ⁿᵈ Trigon of Spiritual Rights – Spirit Halo Chakra

Those in the spirit halo chakra have learned to decide when to accept something and when not to. Depending on your health and medical needs, some foods can be accepted or avoided. Eight guidelines are set forth, and each person aligning the spirit chakra must learn when to use each for nutritive, medicinal, or therapeutic needs. They follow a set of simple guidelines. The guidelines are not mandatory and therefore can be overridden when essential for health.

First Guideline: They avoid all grains (grass seeds) such as rice, corn, and wheat. Pseudocereals are accepted as the seed of a flower. (2 Esdras 12:51) One example of comprehending this spiritual guideline is that if you have difficulty with digestion, a wild rice may be used as a medical need. If you cannot get wild rice, purple rice is a second choice, and red is also a decent choice. Black rice is avoided.

Second Guideline: They don't eat vine foods other than what is needed to complete nutrient or medical and therapeutic needs.

Third Guideline: They avoid ocean, sea, and water plants such as seaweed and watercress. Keep waterways clean and safe for the environment.

Fourth Guideline: Leafy greens such as kale and broccoli are to be avoided for at least 8 days per year around August and September to share with the insects. Greens are added to complete any missing nutrient density and are not the centerpiece of the Livet.

Fifth Guideline: They exclude oils on Wednesdays and Fridays and only use unrefined oils. They may exclude oils altogether if they choose.

Sixth Guideline: Genetically modified foods should be avoided as much as possible. They are not forbidden if the evolution of humanity requires them. Some of the foods that are genetically modified are yellow squash, zucchini, soybeans, corn, papaya, canola, alfalfa, sugar beets, potatoes, arctic apples, rice, and pink pineapples. They are not mandatorily excluded when and if they are the only foods available. Crown chakra wearers are a new species, and we allow divine evolution. Yet if the genetically modified food source has gone to war with farmers and destroyed them, then the crown wearer avoids them to remain in peace.

Seventh Guideline: Organic isn't always the most moral decision. Organic gardening products include bat guano, manure and manure sprays from slaughtered cows, blood, animal gut and egg sprays to deter deer, and ground bone meal. Without these products from farmed animals, organic is the best. With these products, organic is less moral. Organic foods are not mandatory for this reason.

Eighth Guideline: Raw foods should be eaten often. Cooking seeds is a moral decision. Many raw vegans sprout the seeds of foods such as quinoa and eat the new sprouts. This is similar to abortion or killing new life. If a tree were to drop 10,000 seeds, and they all grew right there in one spot, there would be far too many plants; therefore, seeds are obviously designed to be food. Eating sprouted seeds is less moral than eating cooked seeds such as beans. Beans must be cooked after drying, and that is fine. Seeds can have phytic acid, which lowers the intake of certain minerals. If we cook seeds, then we can lower phytic acid to increase the mineral intake of the raw foods that we eat. Prepare foods in the healthiest ways possible.

Many people eat foods that are rough on their bodies and then take vitamins to counteract. That is like putting bad gas in a car every day and then adding a bottle of carburetor and fuel injector cleaner. Acceptable carburetor and fuel injector cleaner has been recommended even with clean gas. Be a healthy and clean, efficient fuel using spiritual organism.

Use the Livet sensibly so that you can connect your physical and spiritual capabilities together and become a spiritual body.

White Ultraviolet 3rd Trigon of Divine Rights – Universal Halo Chakra

Those nutritionally tuned to the universal halo chakra have learned to take care and guard themselves when in need. Those in the universal chakra have aligned their food intake with modern nutritional science so that they can get the best nourishment possible. They make sure that they get 100% of their recommended value of all vitamins and minerals daily, unless otherwise correctly guided. Any needed nutrient which was reduced due to food intake changes can be supplemented. This universal path allows for both science and spirituality to function together. This part of the Livet continues to evolve as research findings assure that the information is modern and correct.

To accomplish the nutritional tuning of the universal chakra, one must prepare to educate others about nutrition and continue learning to take care of everyone.

The 84 Foods

Here is a list of selected foods with numbers. The numbers before the names represent however many vitamins and minerals there are, at 10% daily recommended value or more, in one cup of the listed food. According to science and spirituality, these seem to be the best food choices. The reasoning for this particular selected food list is explained in chapters 9 and 10 of this book.

18: Pistachios
Has low to medium phytic acid.
Level 1 in antioxidants.
Has a calcium level of 11, with great amounts of magnesium, phosphorus, and selenium for bone health.

17: Hazelnuts
Has low phytic acid.
Hazelnut oil has about 4-9% palmitic oil, which makes it a great choice.
Has a calcium level of 2, with a great amount of magnesium for bone health.

17: Pecans
Level 3 in antioxidants.
Has a calcium level of 5, with a great amount of magnesium for bone health.

17: Almonds

Has high phytic acid

Level 2 in antioxidants.

Has a calcium level of 30, with great amounts of magnesium, phosphorus, and selenium for bone health.

Nutritionists recommend eating this food raw in limited amounts and otherwise cooked.

17: Walnuts

Has high phytic acid.

Level 2 in antioxidants.

Has great amounts of magnesium and phosphorus for bone health.

16: Peanuts

Has low to medium phytic acid.

Has great amounts of magnesium, phosphorus, and selenium for bone health.

16: Cashews

Has lectins and/or greater levels of oxalic acid.

Nutritionists recommend eating this food raw in limited amounts and otherwise cooked.

15: Butternut Squash

1 cup = 83% daily value of your vitamin A.

Has a great amount of magnesium for bone health.

15: Macadamia Nuts

Has medium phytic acid.

Has a calcium level of 9, with a great amount of magnesium for bone health.

14: Buckwheat

13: Chia Seeds

Has a great amount of omega 3.

Has lectins and/or greater levels of oxalic acid.

Has a calcium level of 110, with great amounts of magnesium and selenium for bone health.

12: Beans

This food section is for all chosen bean types. Since there are so many kinds of beans that are great for you, only one bean was listed in the 84 foods. The selected beans are in chapter 5 of this book.

12: Sesame Seeds

Level 1 in antioxidants.

Has a great amount of the amino acid methionine for its food category.

Has a calcium level of 23 for bone health.

Nutritionists recommend eating this food raw in limited amounts and otherwise cooked.

12: Coconut

Coconut oil has about 8% palmitic acid, making it a great choice.

Level 2 in antioxidants.

Has a great amount of magnesium and selenium for bone health.

Has medium chain triglycerides.

12: Pumpkin Seeds

Helps increase testosterone.

Has a great amount of the amino acid methionine for its food category.

(9-Pumpkin)

Has lectins and/or greater levels of oxalic acid.

11: Avocados

Avocado oil has about 20% palmitic acid, so avoid it if you can.

Has beneficial lipase enzyme.

Level 3 in antioxidants.

Has a great amount of the amino acid methionine for its food category.

Has great amounts of magnesium, phosphorus, and vitamin K for bone health.

Nutritionists recommend eating this food raw in limited amounts and otherwise cooked. Two small avocados, or one large avocado, is the maximum daily intake.

11: Amaranth (cooked)

Has lectins and/or greater levels of oxalic acid.

Level 2 in antioxidants.

Has a calcium level of 9, with great amounts of magnesium, phosphorus, and selenium for bone health.

11: Acorn Squash

Has a great amount of magnesium for bone health.

10: Quinoa (cooked)

Has lectins and/or greater levels of oxalic acid.

Helps increase testosterone.

Level 2 in antioxidants.

Has a great amount of the amino acid methionine for its food category.

Has a calcium level of 2, with great amounts of magnesium and phosphorus for bone health.

10: Brazil Nuts

Has very high phytic acid.

Has a great amount of the amino acid methionine for its food category.

Has a calcium level of 12 for bone health.

9: Yellow Straightneck Squash

Has lectins and/or greater levels of oxalic acid.

8: Turnip Greens

Level 1 in antioxidants.

Has a calcium level of 8, with a great amount of vitamin K for bone health.

8: Guava

Has a great amount of the amino acid methionine for its food category.

Has a calcium level of 2 for bone health.

8: Okra

Has solanine.

Has a great amount of the amino acid methionine for its food category.

Has a calcium level of 6, with great amounts of magnesium and vitamin K for bone health.

Nutritionists recommend eating this food raw in limited amounts and otherwise cooked.

7: Mango

Has the beneficial amylase enzyme.

7: Kiwi

Has the beneficial protease enzyme.

Has a great amount of the amino acid methionine for its food category.

Has a calcium level of 5, with a great amount of vitamin K for bone health.

7: Celery

Helps increase testosterone.

Has a calcium level of 3, with a great amount of vitamin K for bone health.

7: Asparagus

Has a great amount of the amino acid methionine for its food category.

Has a great amount of vitamin K for bone health.

Nutritionists recommend eating this food raw in limited amounts and otherwise cooked.

7: Red Bell Pepper

Has lectins and/or greater levels of oxalic acid.

Has solanine.

7: Dandelion Greens

Has a calcium level of 8, with a great amount of vitamin K for bone health.

7: Honeyberries

Nutritional information limited. Nutritional value guessed.

6: Brussel Sprouts

Helps remove heavy metals.

Has a great amount of the amino acid methionine for its food category.

Has a calcium level of 3, with a great amount of vitamin K for bone health.

5: Pineapple

Has the beneficial protease and bromelain enzymes.

Has a great amount of the amino acid methionine for its food category.

Has a calcium level of 2 for bone health.

5: Spinach

Helps increase testosterone.

Helps remove heavy metals.

Has lectins and/or greater levels of oxalic acid.

Has a great amount of the amino acid methionine for its food category.

Has a calcium level of 2, with a great amount of vitamin K for bone health.

Nutritionists recommend eating this food raw in limited amounts and otherwise cooked.

5: Cauliflower

Level 2 in antioxidants.

Has a great amount of vitamin K for bone health.

Orange cauliflower is said to have more nutrients.

5: Blackberries

Level 2 in antioxidants.

Has a calcium level of 3, with a great amount of vitamin K for bone health.

5: Bok Choi

Level 1 in antioxidants.

Has a great amount of vitamin K for bone health.

5: Chayote Squash

Has lectins and/or greater levels of oxalic acid.

5: Spondias Mombin

Nutrition facts are limited thus far.

4: Broccoli

Has the beneficial mannose enzyme.

Level 3 in antioxidants.

Has a great amount of the amino acid methionine for its food category.

4: Apricots

Has the beneficial invertase enzyme.

Has a calcium level of 2 for bone health.

4: Chinese Cabbage

Level 2 in antioxidants.

Has a calcium level of 4, with a great amount of vitamin K for bone health.

4: Romaine Lettuce

Level 2 in antioxidants.

Has a great amount of vitamin K for bone health.

4: Lychee

3: Strawberries

Level 2 in antioxidants.

Has a calcium level of 2 for bone health.

3: Red Leaf Lettuce

1 cup = 70% daily value of your vitamin A.

Level 2 in antioxidants.

Has a great amount of vitamin K for bone health.

3: Beet Greens

1 cup = 80% daily value of your vitamin A.

Has lectins and/or greater levels of oxalic acid.

Has a calcium level of 3, with a great amount of vitamin K for bone health.

3: Cabbage

Has the beneficial mannose enzyme.

Level 2 in antioxidants.

Has a calcium level of 3, with a great amount of vitamin K for bone health.

3: Swiss Chard

1 cup = 73% daily value of your vitamin A.

Has lectins and/or greater levels of oxalic acid.

Has a calcium level of 1, with a great amount of vitamin K for bone health.

Nutritionists recommend eating this food raw in limited amounts and otherwise cooked.

3: Mustard Greens

Level 1 in antioxidants.

Has a calcium level of 5, with a great amount of vitamin K for bone health.

3: Mulberries

Has a calcium level of 4 for bone health.

3: Moringa Leaves

Has a calcium level of 240 for bone health.

3: Blueberries

Has beneficial mannose enzyme.

Has solanine.

Level 3 in antioxidants.

Has a great amount of vitamin K for bone health.

3: Collard Greens

Level 2 in antioxidants.

Has a calcium level of 5 for bone health.

3: Green Bell Pepper

Has lectins and/or greater levels of oxalic acid.

Has solanine.

3: Tomato

Has beneficial mannose enzyme.

Has lectins and/or greater levels of oxalic acid.

Has solanine.

Has a great amount of vitamin K for bone health.

3: Ripe Persimmons

3: Rambutan

2: Cherries

Level 2 in antioxidants.

2: Kale

Level 3 in antioxidants.

Has a great amount of the amino acid methionine for its food category.

Has a calcium level of 3, with a great amount of vitamin K for bone health.

2: Peaches

Has beneficial mannose enzyme.

Level 1 in antioxidants.

2: Nectarine

2: Pears

2: Green Beans

Has the beneficial mannose enzyme.

Has lectins and/or greater levels of oxalic acid.

Has a calcium level of 5 for bone health.

Has Iodine

2: Plums

Level 2 in antioxidants.

Nutritionists recommend eating this food raw in limited amounts and otherwise cooked.

2: Prunes

Level 3 in antioxidants.

2: Papaya

Has beneficial protease and papain enzymes.

1: Iceberg Lettuce

Level 2 in antioxidants.

Has a great amount of vitamin K for bone health.

1: Arugula

Level 2 in antioxidants.

Has a calcium level of 2, with a great amount of vitamin K for bone health.

1: Rapini

Has a great amount of vitamin K for bone health.

Selected Spices

Though many spices don't pass the guidelines because of being extra pungent, these few do. Here are some of the herbs highest in antioxidants.

Allspice

Basil

Ceylon Cinnamon
Helps increase testosterone.

Cilantro
Helps remove heavy metals.

Cumin

Holy Basil
Helps remove heavy metals.

Marjoram

Mint

Oregano

Paprika

Mild to medium spiciness

Has solanine.

Black Pepper

Mild spiciness

Sumac

Thyme

Vanilla bean

Eating the Livet doesn't mean that food cannot taste good. It is about not placing flavor before righteousness and health. Enjoy your food. You can find flavors that you like.

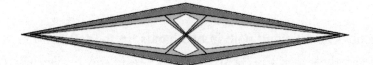

Chapter 5
Sculptor's Diet (Livet)

In this chapter you can find nutritional guidance for those eating from the 84 foods list. The Livet delivers superlative nourishment.

Chartreuse Galactic Stem Chakra of Physical Blessing – Aurora Australis

Those in the chartreuse galactic chakra have completed the entire white trigonal chakra of ascension. They wear their crown of life. They have become enlightened and are ready to educate.

You must be a universal being before you are ready to become galactically aligned. This chakra is beyond universal. Here you can become worthy of your job.

Those in the galactic chakra are ready to head out into the world as professionals. When they do, they may travel and meet with people. They are to be protective of whatever and whomever they come into contact with. They are to be careful with themselves and others. They do their best not to spread bacteria and viruses. They keep their hands clean and/or use hand sanitizer when necessary. When needed, they wear dust masks to guard themselves from bacteria and other debris that could be harmful to the lungs. One recommendation is to have an air purifier to keep the oxygen in their homes clean. If they can, they should wear sunglasses and reef-safe sunscreen to protect their eyes and skin when in prolonged sun exposure. They should drink clean and/or purified water of some kind. They should wear earplugs when coming in contact with loud noises that may damage their ears. While leading by example, those in the chartreuse chakra can help others learn to care for their own health.

The galactic chakra is about educating others on health and being considerate. It is between the yellow solar plexus and the green true heart that people begin turning to kindness. There we find where real compassion is initiated. That's one of the reasons that this chakra is drawn out from the others.

Fish are known to be attracted to the color **chartreuse**. Being in this chakra is similar to being hired to go fishing. (Matthew 4:19) (Mark 1:17) The students are like fish. **The pupils learn better when they are** pescatarian at minimum. This helps ensure that they are receptive to the education.

The galactic chakra functions as a fishing pole in two hands. In the left hand rests the lower heart between the yellow solar plexus and the green true heart. There we find those who are ready to transition beyond pescatarian. In the lower heart, we educate in converting to vegetarian.

In the right hand rests the upper heart between the green and cyan chakras. There the willing students are prepared for their transition beyond vegetarian. We help steady their path so that they can become vegan if they choose. (Matthew 5:41)

(Gnostic Gospel of Truth) "He is the shepherd who left behind the ninety-nine sheep which had not strayed and went in search of that one which was lost. He rejoiced when he had found it. For ninety-nine is a number of the left hand, which holds it. The moment he finds the one, however, the whole number is transferred to the right hand. Thus, it is with him who lacks the one, that is, the entire right hand which attracts that in which it is deficient, seizes it from the left side and transfers it to the right. In this way, then, the number becomes one hundred.

CODEX I Translated by Robert M. Grant From Robert M. Grant, Gnosticism (Harper & Brothers, New York, 1961), as quoted in Willis Barnstone, The Other Bible (Harper & Row, San Francisco, 1984).

To accomplish the nutritional tuning of the galactic chakra, one must educate others about scientifically and spiritually tuning their food intake. They must also help people learn to care for themselves and others.

Optimum Nutritional Training

The Nine Food Groups
1: Beans
2: Berries
3: Tree fruits
4: Fruit 'other'
5: Leafy green vegetables
6: Vegetables 'other"
7: Nuts and seeds
8: Pseudocereals (and grain-type foods)
9: Fats (oils), sodium, supplements

Nutrients and Colors
In the Bible, the throne is depicted as a rainbow like an emerald. This means that we can and should eat all colors of food. (Revelation 4:3) Many nutrients may still be undetected. We can get a variety of the eight colors of foods to help ensure that we obtain these hidden nutrients.

1: Red foods such as cherries

2: Orange foods such as butternut squash

3: Yellow foods such as guava

4: Chartreuse foods such as Chinese cabbage

5: Green foods such as turnip greens

6: Cyan foods such as the bluish broccoli and kale, and certain edible flowers if they can be found

7: Blue foods such as Nona Agnes Blue Beans and certain edible flowers if they can be found

8: Purple foods such as plums and blueberries.

Some foods also come in black, white, brown, and gray. If you have a reason to avoid tannins as much as you can, foods should be selected as white as possible.

93

Recommended Meals for Optimal Nutrition

Once you have entered the chartreuse chakra, you can educate others in ways to align their nutrients. This is done using the 84 foods selected for the Livet.

Those who exercise a lot usually demand the greatest amount of nutrition. To find out how well the Sculptor's Livet can provide, this meal plan was designed for professional bodybuilders.

Meal Type 1: Vitamins C, E, several B vitamins, and potassium can be sensitive to heat, freezing, light, or air. Because of this, a raw blended meal is recommended to increase these nutrients.

Certain nutrients need to conjunct with others so that our bodies can absorb and use them. Blending raw foods keeps all the vitamins and minerals readily available and together for maximum absorption. This Livet suggests eating at least one calcium-rich micronutrient-conjunct meal per day.

Suggested Foods for a Blended Meal:

¾ cup avocado (for lipase enzyme)
1 kiwi (for protease enzyme)
¾ cup pineapple (for protease and bromelain enzymes)
¾ cup mango (for amylase enzyme)
1 celery stalk (for testosterone)
1 ½ cups chopped turnip greens
1 ½ cups chopped kale
1 cup chopped broccoli
1 Brussels sprout (for heavy metal removal)
½ oz chia seeds
1 cup dry roasted peanuts
1 serving of pea protein isolate with (27 grams protein)

Place into a 68 oz blender with water.
Drink with 2 oz of hazelnut oil for extra calories.

This complete meal provides over 1,700 calories and 75 grams of protein to start your day. This combination has well over 100% RDI of each of your essential amino acids. Without the protein isolate, the amino acid lysine drops to about 101% RDI. The blend may include your necessary and/or preferred supplements.

Note from nutritionist. This is an elite meal. It isn't very easy to drink, yet it is wonderful for your health.

Meal Type 2: Pseudocereals for the Livet are selected gluten-free and have great amounts of calcium. These seeds put together form a completeness of protein. With vegan foods, the amino acid methionine can be somewhat restricted. These cereals help increase your methionine.

Quinoa uncooked is said to have about 525 milligrams of methionine per cup.
Amaranth uncooked is said to have about 436 milligrams of methionine per cup.
Two tablespoons of uncooked chia seeds are said to have about 167 milligrams of methionine.

Here is an example mixture for these foods.

Quinoa 12.5 lbs
Amaranth 12.5 lbs
Chia 2 lbs

One raw cup of these mixed cereals can have about 522 milligrams (72% RDI) of methionine. One raw cup of this mixture is a single meal. The recommendation is two of these meals daily. Eating two cups (raw before cooked) twice provides more than 1,400 calories and 53 grams of protein. This combination has well over 100% RDI of each of your essential amino acids.

If this meal is hard to eat when dry after being cooked, like rice, you can boil it. After it cools down a bit, you can add a little water and basically drink the meal.

You may like to add four or five pounds of sesame seeds into the cereal mixture. Sesame seems to pass through undigested. Their hard shells don't open like the other seeds while cooking. Before mixing your cereal, you can get a seed grinder such as the (Vevor 2500g Electric Grain Mill Grinder, 3750W High-Speed Commercial Spice Grinder). Grinding the seeds before mixing the cereals unlocks a powerhouse of nutrients. Sesame seeds are said to have about 1172 milligrams of methionine per cup.

Meal type 3: This daily meal includes two and a half cups of prepared beans, with added vegetables and fresh fruit.

While cooking vegetables causes nutrient loss in some areas, it also provides nutrients in several ways. Cooking certain vegetables reduces antinutrients such as solanine, oxalates, and phytates. It causes some nutrients, such as lycopene and beta-carotene, to become more bioavailable. Cooking vegetables can also help with digestibility.

Here is a list of vegetables that offer different nutrients when cooked: spinach, asparagus, tomatoes, bell peppers, broccoli, cauliflower, celery, green beans, kale, Brussels sprouts, pumpkin, cabbage, beet greens, and butternut squash. Some nutritionists believe that these are better for you when cooked.

Nightshade vegetables can be cooked in coconut oil or hazelnut oil to help reduce the solanine. You can add the nightshades (if you eat them) to the blend of vegetables that are considered better for you when cooked. The Livet calls for a fasting from oils on Wednesdays and Fridays. Because of this fasting, nightshades could also at least be avoided on these days. Vegetables are steamed instead of stir-fried on Wednesdays and Fridays. Beans are added to the cooked meal.

Beans for the Livet are selected for their great amounts of calcium and methionine while having lower contents of purines. Five primary beans have been chosen based on these guidelines. The numbers before the names represent however many vitamins and minerals there are, at 10% daily recommended value or more, per one cup of the listed bean.

9: Cranberry Beans Cooked
7% daily calcium per cup
About 248 milligrams of methionine per cup

13: Pink Beans Cooked
7% daily calcium per cup
About 230 milligrams of methionine per cup

11: Black Beans Cooked
4% daily calcium per cup
About 229 milligrams of methionine per cup
Said to have high levels of antioxidants.

12: Black Turtle Beans Cooked

8% daily calcium per cup

About 228 milligrams of methionine per cup

14: Navy Beans Cooked

10% daily calcium per cup

About 202 milligrams of methionine per cup

Example Dinner

Place these into a pan and lightly fry them together. You could add a little water to soften the vegetables. (Steam them on Wednesdays and Fridays instead of stir-frying.)

1 tbsp coconut oil

1 celery stalk

1 cup butternut squash

½ cup tomatoes

¾ cup chopped bell pepper

1 cup red cabbage

Next, add these raw ingredients to the stir-fried veggies.

½ cup blueberries

¾ cup strawberries

¾ cup avocado

1 cup romaine lettuce

2 ½ cups cranberry beans

This meal contains about 725 milligrams (100% RDI) of methionine. The recommendation is to eat one of these meals daily. It provides over 1,250 calories and 54 grams of protein. This combination has 100% RDI or more of each of your essential amino acids. You can exclude the cooked vegetables if you choose.

Daily Nutritional Value

Here are the nutritional values if all four of these meals are eaten daily.

Information resourced from https://www.myfooddata.com/

Macronutrients

Calories: 4,401 – 220% DV

Carbohydrates: 534g – 194% DV

Fat: 196g – 251% DV

Fiber: 134g – 480% DV

Protein: 181g – 362% DV

Sugar: 82g – 165% DV

Micronutrients – Minerals and Vitamins

A Vitamin RAE: 246% DV

B1 Thiamin: 265% DV

B2 Riboflavin: 213% DV

B3 Niacin: 267% DV

B5 Pantothenic Acid: 259% DV

B6 Pyridoxine: 328% DV

B9 Folate: 628% DV

Beta Carotene: 216% DV

C Vitamin: 762% DV

Calcium: 128% DV

Choline: 93% DV is listed. This value has missing data on several foods. The actual DV is over 100%.

Copper Cu: 643% DV

E Vitamin: 300% DV

Iron Fe: 270% DV

K1 Vitamin: 916% DV

Magnesium: 409% DV

Manganese: 826% DV

Phosphorus, P: 303% DV

Potassium, K: 205% DV

Selenium Se: 176% DV

Zinc Zn: 237% DV

Amino Acid Profile

Cystine: 769% RDI

Histidine: 684% RDI

Isoleucine: 524% RDI

Leucine: 463% RDI

Lysine: 489% RDI

Methionine: 374% RDI

Phenylalanine: 1,005% RDI

Threonine: 647% RDI

Tryptophan: 757% RDI

Tyrosine: 614% RDI

Valine: 471% RDI

This meal plan was designed for specialized bodybuilding. The nutrient totals include one supplement of pea protein isolate. Adding an extra serving of pea protein brings the value to over 200 grams daily. According to research, that amount of protein should be enough for a lean, muscular 200- to 285-lb man. If more is needed, pea isolate can be increased.

Meal type 4: A snack meal with fruit and seeds or nuts can be added if desired. Raw butternut squash is highly recommended daily.

Secondary Choice Beans

These four beans have less methionine or other nutrients, yet are acceptable.

12: Kidney Beans Cooked

5% daily calcium per cup

About 200 milligrams of methionine per cup

Has Mannose Enzyme

Said to have high levels of antioxidants

13: Pinto Beans Cooked

6% daily calcium per cup

About 200 milligrams of methionine per cup

Said to have high levels of antioxidants

Small Red Beans Cooked

7% daily calcium per cup

Missing nutrition information.

Chosen for very high levels of antioxidants

Nona Agnes' Blue Beans Cooked

Missing nutrition information.

Chosen for blue flavonoids

Fasting Plan

While bodybuilders require a lot of food, some people prefer to eat fewer calories. The Livet is versatile and offers a yearly fasting plan. Doing your fasting this way opens blessings from GOD.

It is said that fasting can reduce inflammation and aging to extend your life span. It may also help get rid of many illnesses. It may increase mental, heart, and digestive health. It can also cleanse the body and help with various forms of obesity.

This fasting isn't for pushing the body into suffering; it is to be conducive to good health. The various fasting guidelines in the Livet have been put together in a way that works well and doesn't harm the body. Depending on health and location, some people cannot fast from water. Water can be consumed on any fasting day for health needs. You may do all of these or even just those you choose. Supplementing vitamins and minerals during fasting days if medically required.

Fasting Rules

January 3rd from sunrise to sunset – (without food and drink)

Jan 5th – (eat only raw vegetables, nuts, and fruits without oil)

January 6th – (only eat after noon)

January 6th to December 25th – (on all Fridays, eat only raw vegetables, nuts, and fruits without oil)

Feb 22nd to April 7th – (eat only two meals without oil, yet on Wednesdays and Fridays eat only one meal)

February 26th – (eat only until noon)

March 1st – (eat only two meals either before or after noon)

March 2nd to 20th – (be without food and drink while the sun is up)

March 3rd – (eat only two meals either before or after noon)

March 5th – (without food and drink from sunrise to sunset)

March 9th – (eat only raw vegetables, nuts, and fruits without oil)

March 22nd to April 20th – (be without food and drink while the sun is up)

March 26th – (eat only raw vegetables, nuts, and fruits, without oil)

April 6th – (don't eat food after noon)

April 7th – (fast from food for 24 hours)

May 28th – (eat only raw vegetables, nuts, and fruits without oil)

May 29th to June 4th – (be without food and drink while the sun is up)

June 5th to June 29th – (eat only raw vegetables, nuts, and fruits without oil)

July 6th – (without food and drink from sunrise to sunset)

July 26th at sunset to the 27th at sunset plus one hour – (without food and drink for 25 hours)

August 14th to 23rd – (without green vegetables and don't eat after sunset)

August 1st to 15th – (eat only raw vegetables, nuts, and fruits without oil. Eat only two meals on the second Wednesday and Friday – Wednesday and Friday meals should be eaten before or after noon)

August 29th – (eat only raw vegetables, nuts, and fruits without oil)

September 14th – (eat only raw vegetables, nuts, and fruits without oil)

September 18th – (without food and drink from sunrise to sunset)

September 24th at sunset to the 25th at sunset – (without food and drink)

Extra Fasting Rules if Needed

On one day per week, on any day, don't eat after noon.

On the first Sunday of each month, don't eat or drink. This is done from sundown on Saturday till sundown on Sunday (24 hours). The resources that you save can go to feed those in need. A small donation is set aside each month when doing this.

Miscellaneous Livetary Tips

1: Natural salts are known to have heavy metals. It is said that Lake Deborah Sea Salt doesn't have any heavy metals, and if so, this salt is great for sodium intake. Some of the other salts that have been said to have tested the lowest in heavy metals are Diamond Crystal Kosher Salt, Maldon Sea Salt Flakes, and Saltverk Flaky Sea Salt.

2: Iodized salt isn't included in the Livet. Some iodine can be found in green beans, strawberries, and prunes. Deep-earth-sourced iodine is the recommended supplement.

3: Using a sweetener isn't needed. Blended fruits are the recommendation. If any sweetener is used, the recommendation is coconut sugar.

4: Coconuts are a great source of medium-chain triglycerides.

5: Coconut is said to be good for the lungs.

6: The recommended oils are hazelnut oil and coconut oil. Palmitic acid is said to shorten telomeres. Hazelnut oil has very low palmitic acid compared to other oils. Research states that the lauric acid in coconut doesn't shorten telomeres.

7: Olives have the most hydroxytyrosol, which may be the strongest antioxidant known, yet the tree can have thorns. Olives from thornless olive trees are acceptable.

8: Herbs are acceptable. The suggestion is that we don't use strong spices in extremes which drastically change the flavor. This way we can acquire the new taste, that doesn't enable us to choose flavor over health. If your mind isn't choosing flavor over health, then it rewires the synapse to enjoy healing rather than to enjoy damaging stimulations.

9: When using frozen fruits for blended meals, fruits that have been peeled before freezing them are better for you. Unpeeled fruits may have more pesticides. Peeled fruits will be cleaner and don't have to be washed as fruits that have peels do.

10: If you eat peanuts, including the red skins provides beneficial resveratrol. You may also grind your peanuts and drink them in blended meals. Blended nuts should present a greater nutrient bioavailability.

11: Though sunflower seeds are not on the list of foods to consume, you may supplement with sunflower lecithin or other types of lecithin if you choose.

12: The protease enzyme in kiwi, pineapple, and papaya is systemic and enters the entire body.

13: Amaranth is considered the food of the divine. Holy Basil is considered holy. Moringa is called the Miracle Tree and the Tree of Immortality. Each of these is acceptable. Together they are three special keys.

14: It has been said that boiling pseudocereals does not reduce much of the needed Omega-3.

15: Butternut squash is recommended every day, especially raw.

16: Kiwi, avocado, guava, pineapple, Brussels sprouts, spinach, asparagus, okra, broccoli, and kale have more methionine than most foods in their food groups.

17: Hazelnuts, pistachios, and peanuts each have decent methionine levels. They are also lower in phytic acid than most other seeds and nuts. Macadamia nuts may also be lower in phytic acid than many others.

18: Pressure cooking beans can make them easier to digest. It is said that pressure cooking breaks down complex fibers, reduces indigestible sugars by more than 75%, removes most of the anti-nutrients, and allows for the absorption of more iron. Some people recommend soaking the beans for 8-12 hours before rinsing and cooking. Suggestions include placing beans in a pressure cooker with water 2" above the beans. Use high pressure or 15 lbs, and cook for 10-12 minutes. Times and pressure may vary depending on altitude and bean of choice.

19: There are two primary types of bean protein isolates: soy and pea. Many people are allergic to soy. A lot of beans, such as peas, have low methionine. The best bean protein isolates would seem to be from cranberry, pink, black, or black turtle beans.

20: You can add raw fruit to any meal for increasing nutrients and flavor.

21: Whenever we see an organic food next to a genetically modified food, choosing the organic version can reduce pesticide use and pollution. Yet buying organic can increase the use of animal products.

22: Manufactured foods such as noodles and breads, as long as they have no other ingredients, are basically considered safe. This includes foods such as bean noodles that only have the bean as an ingredient. The worst component of these foods may be the packaging, which can be recycled.

23: When eating plant-based foods, the best thing to eat is that which you grow yourselves.

24: Foods that you have canned yourself at home in jars without chemical preservatives are acceptable.

25: The mushrooms that have the most vitamin D2 are penny bun, maitake, morel, and chanterelle in order. These mushrooms grow on forest beds by trees and don't thrive on manure. Growing them in a sterile environment to extract vitamin D2 isn't prohibited.

26: Carnivorous plants such as figs, oyster mushrooms, and shaggy mane mushrooms should not be eaten nor used for supplements. These plants are meat eaters. Vegans should avoid meat-eating plants.

27: Only purified water is recommended for ingesting. Reverse osmosis and faucet filtration systems can help. Alkaline systems are also recommended. Some water filters, such as ultrafiltration, are said to remove bacteria and viruses. Some people boil their water to clean it, yet that doesn't filter it.

28: Get a little bit of sunlight, yet not so much that it increases aging. If you are going to be in the sun a lot, go ahead and put on some vegan reef-safe sunscreen. Find something that isn't going to harm the atmosphere and the water supply. Also wear some sunglasses to protect yourselves from ultraviolet light if you will be outside in bright lights for a length of time. If you are going to be using electronics such as computers often, put some blue light-blocking glasses on to protect your eyes.

29: Feel your body. Move and express in the ways that you desire. Does your body crave motion? Doing things like running, walking, exercising, yoga, and dancing allows your body to move in ways that it wants and needs.

30: Plant protein is said to be better for the kidneys than animal-based products.

31: The Livet is designed to help produce a healthy intestinal microbiome. It is in our hopes that you can begin producing B12 in your small intestines, where it is absorbed. You may need the mineral cobalt, which is in nuts and leafy greens, to do this. Leafy greens should have enough cobalt to perform the necessary needs to help produce B12 if you can.

32: The most common vegan food allergies are seeds, peanuts, tree nuts, soy, wheat, and corn. If you have a problem converting to veganism, and it is making you sick, then your first option is to check for reactions to these foods.

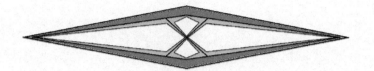

Chapter 6
Divine Gateway

Divine Gateway of Nutrition

To enter the divine gateway chakra of nutritional intake, one must follow every advanced rule of the Livet.

When plants offer fruits and seeds, you cannot be considered stealing for eating them. Plants willingly help us. Fruits and whole-fruit vegetables were designed for you to eat. They are provided as food.

Though the plants willingly give food, taking leaves could be considered stealing if they were not granted to us. For this reason, as well as others, some Jains don't eat the leaves of plants.

Here are the details of why.

Research shows that plants can both talk and hear. If you cut a plant, the plant speaks or even screams. They can perceive when insects chew them. Adding to this reasoning, research shows that plants can also learn and remember. These next three links have information on these subjects. (Psalm 96:12)

https://english.tau.ac.il/plants_emit_sounds

https://www.snexplores.org/article/plants-listen-danger

https://en.wikipedia.org/wiki/Plant_cognition

Rule One: Here is a list of plants that could be considered stolen from for food.

Arugula
Asparagus
Basil
Beet Greens
Bok Choy
Broccoli
Brussels Sprouts
Cabbage
Cauliflower
Celery
Ceylon Cinnamon
Chinese Cabbage
Cilantro
Collard Greens
Dandelion Greens
Holy Basil
Iceberg Lettuce
Kale
Marjoram
Mint
Moringa Leaves
Mustard Greens
Oregano
Rapini
Red Leaf Lettuce
Romaine Lettuce
Spinach
Swiss Chard
Thyme
Turnip Greens

Rule Two: Some plants are cut to harvest their seeds. Because of this, these plants can be considered stolen from for food as well. If the harvester gathers the seeds without harming the plant, then the seeds are not considered stolen.

Rule Three: While seeds are provided and given by the plants as food, some Jains recommend not eating seeds or many-seed fruits. This list includes foods that some Jains would avoid because of the number of seeds. Peanuts could also be avoided because they grow underground. This list includes foods in rules two and three.

Allspice
Almonds
Amaranth
Beans
Blackberries
Black Pepper
Brazil Nuts
Buckwheat
Cashews
Chia Seeds
Coconut
Cumin
Guava
Hazelnuts
Honeyberries
Macadamia Nuts
Mulberries
Papaya
Peanuts
Pears
Pecans
Persimmons
Pineapple
Pistachios
Quinoa
Sesame Seeds
Strawberries
Sumac
Vanilla bean
Walnuts

Rule Four: Some Rastas recommend avoiding eating from vine plants. Here is a list of foods that they would avoid. These also fit into rule three.

Acorn Squash
Butternut Squash
Chayote Squash
Green Beans
Kiwi
Pumpkin and Seeds
Yellow Straightneck Squash

Many or most beans also come from vines.

Rule Five: Some scientific research has guided nutritionist to avoid foods with solanine. Here is a list of foods that have solanine. These also fit into rule three.

Blueberries
Green Bell Pepper
Okra
Paprika
Red Bell Pepper
Tomato

Twelve Fruits of Life

Some Jains recommend only eating plants with the least seeds possible and to not eat seeds at all. When this rule is followed, along with all others, there are only 12 foods remaining of the 84. Each of these foods must have only one seed, which isn't the food portion of the fruit. These twelve foods stand the test of every nutrition regulation found.

These are twelve fully approved fruits of the Tree of Life. These foods have passed every test possible through both religion and science. They are especially good for fruit fasting and cleansing days. You can also eat and drink from these fruits when sick. (2 Esdras 2:14-19)

These twelve foods are considered heavenly. These fruits and their juices are the ambrosia and nectar that the ancient Greeks spoke about.

Apricots
Avocados
Cashew Apples
Cherries
Lychee
Mango
Nectarine
Peaches
Plums
Prunes
Rambutan
Spondias Mombin

If we could survive on just these fruits, that would be great. Since we cannot survive healthfully without complete nutrition at this moment, all 84 foods have been approved from heaven. If we find a way to survive with only the 12 foods mentioned here, that would be perfect. If you cannot survive on these foods alone, you can add in the seeds in the list of foods. This is allowed because we know that not all seeds can be planted, and therefore not eating them could be considered a waste of resources.

Unlocking the Path to the Tree of Life

Long ago the path to the tree of life was blocked. A flaming sword had been placed in the way to guard the tree. The sword turned in every direction.

To find the tree of life, we must find the flaming sword. It is the mouths of religious leaders and followers. (Psalm 57:4, 64:3) (Hosea 7:16) Leaders pointed their tongues like swords at one another. There were so many houses arguing that their words turned every way. They devoured each other. (Baruch 3:9-14)

This fiery sword was there to deter the belief that the religions all came from GOD. Each word was harsh. Flaming mouths made hearts sick for loss of hope. (Proverbs 13:12) (Baruch 3:15-28)

To get to the tree of life, the people must listen to a wholesome tongue. (Proverbs 15:4) GOD placed the keys of the tree into many religions. They were all part of one body. A single sword had turned against itself. It is time for them to congratulate one another for each having something incredible from GOD.

Together they are a righteous kingdom from heaven. The entirety of these religions is one child, the fruit of the righteous. (Proverbs 11:30)

Open the path by connecting religious keys with science. Paradise of GOD becomes opened. (Revelation 2:7)

The Heavenly Mother, the Holy Ghost, has delivered them. (Proverbs 3:18) She is also known as Wisdom and Jerusalem from above. (James 3:17) (Galatians 4:26) (2 Esdras 2:10, 2:15, 2:30, 13:36) (Baruch 3:29-37)

As you can see, by following the guidance of all religions and science together, the path is found. More about the alignments and path to the tree of life is found in chapters 10 and 11 of this book.

The Livet is the Tree of Life in food form. Eating it doesn't guarantee that you will live within your current physical body forever. What it does is provide the changes in the mental synapse of humanity for them as a collective to live forever. The righteousness and obedience to GOD through eating the Livet can also get you sealed in heaven. In that it can provide eternal life.

The author of this book descended into dangerous trials to get the seals and keys of this doctrine. The Livet is what saved his life after the tests he endured. He would have died otherwise.

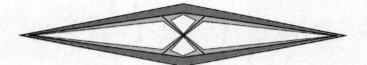

Chapter 7
Bodybuilding Spirituality

Chapters 4 through 6 of this book have revealed how to eat like Christ. This chapter teaches ways to build the body of Christ upon you through exercise.

Decagain

The type of weightlifting recommended is called Decagain. It is a cycle designed to keep an equilibrium with maximum muscle gain and minimum joint stress. Exercises are fit into a five-day workout session, with two days off.

To educate about Decagain, several graphs have been provided. The first graph shows ten sections of the upper body. The right side of the graph has the angles of the front of the body with pushing exercises. The left side of the graph has the angles of the back of the body with pulling exercises. Pull exercises include biceps and shoulder flys. Biceps are in the front, yet are for pulling like back muscle groups. Shoulder flys are for pulling the arms up without pushing on the elbows.

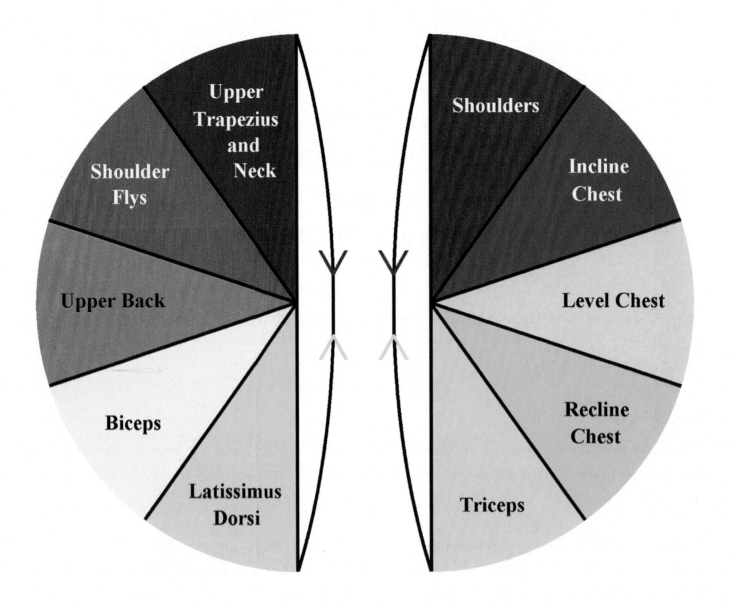

Looking at the first graph, you can see how both the front and back of the body each have five angles of exercise. In the center, there are two purple and chartreuse arrows. Those arrows mean that the chartreuse and purple sections come together on each side. Doing this would make two circles (or stars) with five sections each.

The next graph has two five-pointed stars. Many people learned how to draw a five-point star as a child. Drawing stars is done with straight lines, skipping one point each time until the fifth line reconnects to the beginning point. The exercises are numbered, like drawing a star. The appendages are counted from one to five, beginning with the triceps and upper trapezius and neck, then counterclockwise from there. This makes two Pentagain systems for the front and back of your upper body.

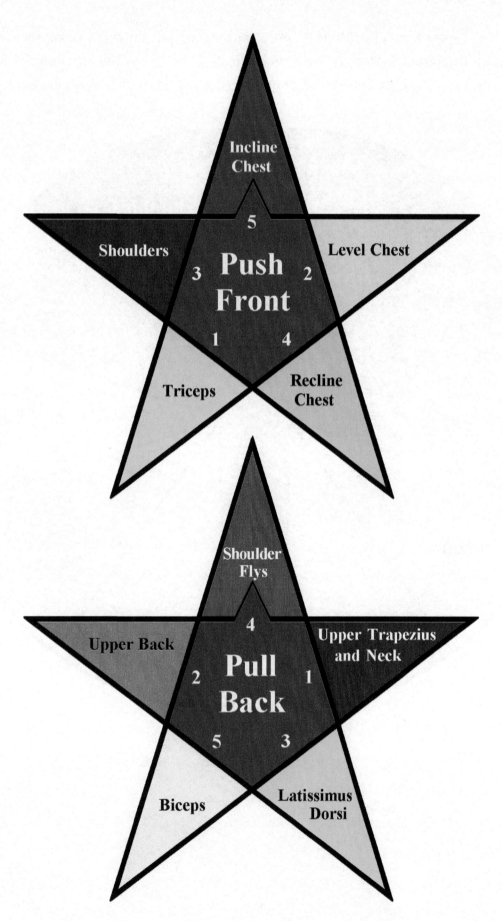

Next, the stars are reopened and placed side by side. The numbers one through five are for Monday through Friday. This means that on day 1-Monday, the exercises include the triceps and upper trapezius and neck. On day 2-Tuesday, the exercises include level chest and upper back. And so on through the week.

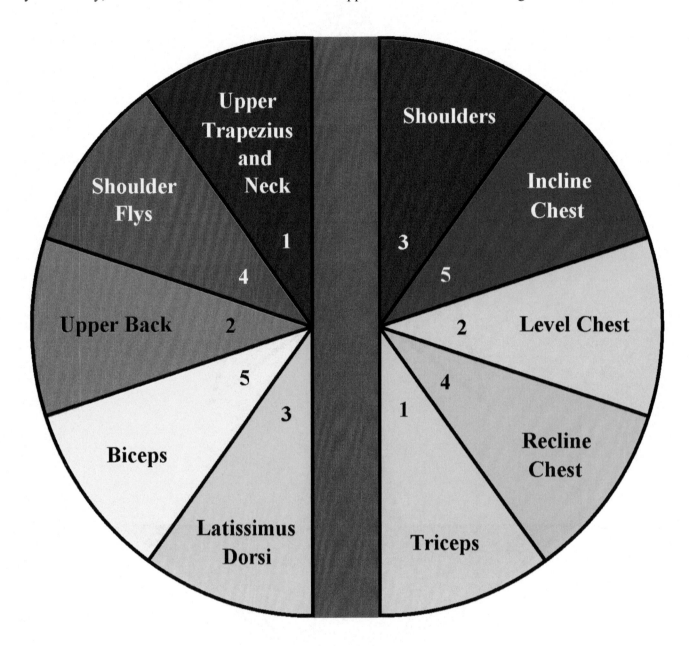

Finally, the back and pulling exercises are numbered after the front and pushing exercises. This brings the dual Pentagain systems into one Decagain routine. The next graph expresses the Decagain.

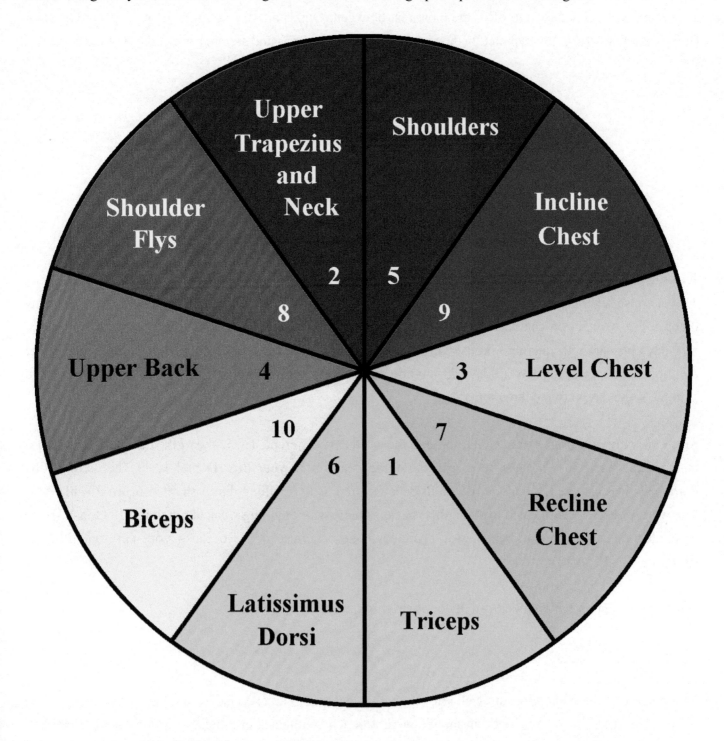

This Decagain approach was designed using the Urim. That is the reason for the colors.

Legs

Leg exercises are added in with their own routine. The torso is included with the legs. Squats and core-back are separated by three days to offer the most rest between. Quads are placed in the center on Wednesdays. Calves and hamstrings are included in the remaining days. Forearms and stomach are entered twice per cycle.

Monday – Glutes (and forearms)
Tuesday – Calves (and stomach)
Wednesday – Quads (and forearms)
Thursday – Hamstrings (and stomach)
Friday – Core Back

Four Strength Quarter Cycles

This exercise schedule has four strength quarters. The strength quarters are lists of guidelines. There are many other exercises that you can do with each muscle group. The recommendation is to lift weights for three to five days per strength quarter. Choose your muscle groups from the lists. You can do some or all of the mentioned exercises. If you skip days during one quarter, leave those exercises behind. Do your best not to skip the same day(s) two quarters in a row.

Since this way of lifting is from GOD, some of the words are different. The name of the deadlift exercise was changed to 'stand-ups' because there isn't anything dead about your lift. (Daniel 12:1) The name of the dumbbells was changed to bells or handbells because there isn't anything dumb about your lift. (Mark 9:25) The word week(s) was changed to strength(s) because there isn't anything weak about your lift. (Job 4:3) The word decline, as in decline bench, was changed to descent/descending because your spiritual lift isn't declining. (Esther 6:13)

Most of the exercises mentioned can be found on this site link.

https://strengthlevel.com/

While many of these exercises are well known, one isn't. There is an exercise in strength three called incline giants. This exercise is done with an incline weight bench (without a bar rack). It is similar to a handbell lateral raise while laying back in the incline position. Begin with your palms facing down and your arms hanging perpendicular with the floor. Do a lateral raise, keeping your palms facing down as long as you can. As you raise your arms, rotate your palms up and bring the bells together above you. Turn your palms back down as you lower your arms. Your arms should hang perpendicular from the ground. This exercise is also called Angel Wings.

116

Strength #1

Monday – (Traps) – Barbell Shrugs

Monday – (Gluts & Quads) – Squats

Monday – (Triceps) – Tricep Dips

Monday – (Forearms) – Hand Grips and/or Grip Twists such as Wrist Curls

Tuesday – (Upper Back) – Bench Pull

Tuesday – (Stomach) – Weighted Hanging Leg Raises

Tuesday – (Calves) – Sitting Calf Raises

Tuesday – (Level Chest) – Reverse Bench Press

Wednesday – (Lats) – Close & Wide Grip Pullups & Lat Pulldowns

Wednesday (Quads) – Leg Extension

Wednesday – (Shoulders) – Behind the Neck Press (Barbell)

Wednesday – (Forearms) – Hand Grips and/or Grip Twists such as Wrist Curls

Thursday – (Shoulder Flys) – Standing Shoulder Fly (all the way above head)

Thursday – (Hemstrings) – Seated Leg Curls

Thursday – (Stomach) – Sit Ups

Thursday – (Lower Chest) – Descending Handbell Bench Press

Friday – (Biceps) – Reverse Barbell Preacher Curl

Friday – (Torso) – Back Extensions

Friday – (Incline Chest) – Incline Bench Press

Friday (Cardio) – Jog

Bodybuilding is very spiritual. Being absorbed in attentiveness to your health can evolve into guidance towards the well-being of others.

Strength #2

Monday – (Traps) – Handbell Shoulder Shrugs

Monday – (Gluts & Quads) – Leg Press (or Squats)

Monday – (Triceps) – Laying Tricep Extension

Monday – (Forearms) – Hand Grips and/or Grip Twists such as Wrist Curls

Tuesday – (Upper Back) – Bent-Over Shoulder Flys

Tuesday – (Stomach) – Weighted Hanging Leg Raises

Tuesday – (Calves) – Standing Calf Raises

Tuesday – (Level Chest) – Bench Press

Wednesday – (Lats) – Pull Ups & Lat Pulldowns – Chin Ups

Wednesday – (Quads) – Leg Extension

Wednesday – (Shoulders) – Seated Handbell Shoulder Press

Wednesday – (Forearms) – Hand Grips and/or Grip Twists such as Wrist Curls

Thursday – (Shoulder Flys) – Barbell Front Raise

Thursday – (Hemstrings) – Seated Leg Curl

Thursday – (Stomach) – Sit Ups

Thursday – (Lower Chest) – Descending Reverse Bench Press

Friday – (Biceps) – Sitting and Standing Hammer Curl

Friday – (Torso) – Stand Ups (previously deadlift)

Friday – (Incline Chest) – Chest Fly

Friday – (Cardio) – Bicycle Ride

Increased physical strength can be very beneficial. You can make sure that your strength is being used in helpful ways. One way is digging holes for planting trees.

Strength #3

Monday – (Traps) – Barbell Shrugs

Monday – (Gluts & Quads) – Squats

Monday – (Triceps) – Tricep Dips

Monday – (Forearms) – Hand Grips and/or Grip Twists such as Wrist Curls

Tuesday – (Upper Back) – Bench Pull

Tuesday – (Stomach) – Weighted Hanging Leg Raises

Tuesday – (Calves) – Sitting Calf Raises

Tuesday – (Level Chest) – Chest Fly

Wednesday – (Lats) – Close & Wide Grip Pullups & Lat Pulldowns

Wednesday (Quads) – Leg Extension

Wednesday – (Shoulders) – Reverse Shoulder Press

Wednesday – (Forearms) – Hand Grips and/or Grip Twists such as Wrist Curls

Thursday – (Shoulder Flys) – Incline Giants & Forward Shoulder Lifts

Thursday – (Hemstrings) – Seated Leg Curls

Thursday – (Stomach) – Sit Ups

Thursday – (Lower Chest) – Descending Bench Press

Friday – (Biceps) – Preacher Curl

Friday – (Torso) – Back Extensions

Friday – (Incline Chest) – Incline Handbell Bench Press

Friday (Cardio) – Jog

Bodybuilding is a very spiritual job which helps you learn symmetry with your surroundings. Be at peace between your sets.

Strength #4

Monday – (Traps) – Behind the Back Barbell Shrugs

Monday – (Gluts & Quads) – Leg Press (or Squats)

Monday – (Triceps) – Handbell Tricep Extension

Monday – (Forearms) – Hand Grips and/or Grip Twists such as Wrist Curls

Tuesday – (Upper Back) – Bent over Row

Tuesday – (Stomach) – Weighted Hanging Leg Raises

Tuesday – (Calves) – Standing Calf Raises

Tuesday – (Level Chest) – Handbell Bench Press

Wednesday – (Lats) – Close Grip Pull Ups & Pulldowns - Chin-ups

Wednesday – (Quads) – Leg Extension

Wednesday – (Shoulders) – Standing Shoulder Press

Wednesday – (Forearms) – Hand Grips and/or Grip Twists such as Wrist Curls

Thursday – (Shoulder Flys) – Handbell Lateral Raise

Thursday – (Hemstrings) – Sitting Leg Curls

Thursday – (Stomach) – Sit Ups

Thursday – (Lower Chest) – Descending Handbell Fly

Friday – (Biceps) – Barbell Curl

Friday – (Torso) – Stand Ups (previously deadlift)

Friday – (Incline Chest) – Reverse Incline Bench Press

Friday – (Cardio) – Bicycle Ride

Exercising can impact your surroundings. Using healthy choices to lead by example can ripple an impact on the health of the entire world. Grab your Rod of Iron and lift.

What Causes Joint Damage

Research has revealed that lifting weights too heavy for doing eight or more reps may harm cartilage. This is due to inflammation and a possible release of chemicals that attack the joints. The same research suggests that exercise with weights that can be lifted for 15-20 reps can prevent damage and enhance cartilage reconstruction.

Here is a link to research on this subject.

https://www.muscleandfitness.com/flexonline/training/build-muscle-mass-while-preventing-joint-damage/

High-impact motion can also harm your cartilage. This includes things such as jumping from very high places and incorrectly landing on your feet. Movements like that can compress and possibly tear your joints.

Can Cartilage be Rebuilt

Research has shown that making small injuries in the cartilage had prompted it to rebuild. Here is a link to research that suggests this possibility.

https://med.stanford.edu/news/all-news/2020/08/Researchers-find-method-to-regrow-cartilage-in-the-joints.html

The problem with that method was that the new cartilage resembles scar tissue. The scar tissue wasn't as strong as the original cartilage, yet it was better than nothing.

Another research suggests that weightlifters who consistently compress their joints have thicker cartilage than those who are physically inactive. This is due to two reasons. First, when we are inactive, the body breaks down any non-used parts. Similar to atrophy, where muscle breaks down when we don't exercise, cartilage may also break down when it isn't used. Second, elite weightlifters program their joints to constantly grow due to the pseudo-injuries to their cartilage.

Jogging is said to cause moderate impacts that can also help with cartilage conditioning and growth in the knees.

Here are two links to sites with research suggesting this possibility.

https://pubmed.ncbi.nlm.nih.gov/24648385/

https://www.wellandgood.com/how-to-build-knee-cartilage/

How does the Livet Help

The research noted can be combined with the nutritional intake of the Sculptors Livet. With this information infused, a healing procedure is revealed.

What we have learned is that when heavy weight is lifted in very low reps, the joints could become inflamed. The body may then react to the swelling by removing some of the cartilage. This process is like the body ignorantly blaming the wrong part of itself. That is comparable to prejudice. The real problem in this portrayal should be seen as the muscles being too strong for the joints. When strength injures joints, the body should know to reduce muscle or otherwise grow the joints.

Why does the body do those things?

It can be hard for certain types of healing to occur due to the simple fact that a hand cannot hear a foot, nor can a shin see the ears, and so on. Without proper communication, the problem can be interpreted incorrectly.

How can these obstacles of inflammation and communication be overcome?

The nourishment of the Livet is in a category of its own. First, eating the Sculptor's Livet can reduce and/or eliminate inflammation in the joints. This is valuable when lifting very heavy.

Second, the Livet instructs the body to regenerate the central nervous system. It has a combination of foods and directions that modify the synapse of the mind. This change allows each part of the body to see and hear one another and therefore communicate. The nervous system can then speak for the joints. It helps stop your internal systems from being confused. The body learns not to blame the incorrect part of itself. You may be required to eat the Livet for a few years before this process can solidify. The Livet was tested for over two years before this book was released.

Once the body parts are transversed, each portion can correspond with one another. Healing can receive a manifold increase. (Mark 5:34) (Acts 14:9)

Rebuilding through Health

It is taught that cartilage continually grows and heals through all ages. Though true, limited blood flow causes it to grow very slowly. Sometimes the rate of growth can occur slower than damage. When joints are injured faster than they heal, they can become depleted.

Nutrients pass through blood vessel walls. When eating meats and dairy products from animals, the intake of cholesterol can further limit nutrient distribution. Too much cholesterol can restrict and/or destroy capillaries and nutrient delivery. Being vegan cleans the vascular system and increases blood flow. Cartilage can grow faster, helping provide sustainable and renewable joints.

Along with excellent blood flow, healthy bones are also needed. Bones feed the joints. This Sculptors Livet is founded on building cartilage through a strong skeletal structure. The main micronutrients needed to build bone density are calcium, vitamin D3, iodine, vitamin K, magnesium, manganese, phosphorus, potassium, selenium, and silica. Eating the Livet correctly makes sure that each of these nutrients is adequately provided. Where there are significant amounts of these nutrients, the bones can begin healing and increasing in density. When the bones have more than enough for just themselves, they can then maintain the cartilage.

With a healthy vascular system and strong bones, the path of nutrients is provided to the cartilage. With strong cartilage, the body can then sustain motion. Remaining in motion helps keep the body alive and thriving while yearning for the nutrients. The more nutrients that the body desires, the more that it is willing to eat. Eating adequate dense nutrients provides availability for building with. Youth endures.

Consistent exercise keeps the vessels open and healthy. They carry sufficient nutrients for healing. When the body has enough, it can send signals through the nerves to measure the health of each joint, bone, and other parts of the body. The mind can even measure the length of limbs and the distance between bones by measuring cartilage tension on nerves. By doing this, the body can then make adjustments.

Rebuilding through Exercise

Your energy is like a muscle. You must use the energy you have to be able to produce more than you previously had. For those who are just beginning, cardio exercises such as light jogging and the elliptical are suggested. Practice increasing your heart rate for 30 minutes. This will begin the muscle toning, fat loss, and energy building.

Get to the point where you can withstand cardio exercises. Then it is time to add in weight training. Lifting weights builds muscle and increases the rate of fat burning. Continue cardio and weightlifting based on your needs. Light to moderate pressure and impact exercises increase bone density and build cartilage.

When lifting weights and pressing hard on the joints, the body may feel like it has been injured though it hasn't. The goal is to cause the body to promote cartilage growth due to pseudo-injuries. In this, the body responds as if it has an injury when it doesn't. Instead of telling the mind that the joints are damaged, train the mind to hear what the joints need.

After heavy lifting without real injury, we can find the mind and body signaling to perform decompression restoration. This allows the strengthening of joints after being compressed. During the process, cartilage grows stronger and thicker.

The goal in weightlifting for longevity is to hold most or all of your heavy sets within the 15-20 rep range. That way you can keep your cartilage in a productive state.

If you must lift heavier to gain muscle, you can use progressive load and bring some sets into the lower rep range. Make sure that your first two or more sets are in the 15-20 rep range. That pre-stimulates the reconstructive tendency in your joints.

Research has revealed that muscle growth tapers off with sets in reps below five. Because of this, we should keep our heaviest sets between the reps of five and eight. If you still cannot grow and choose to bring the rep range below five, make sure that you are fully warmed up before doing so.

When completing an exercise, bring two or more sets back into the 15-20 rep range. This restimulates reconstruction. Each time your joints experience heavy compression, the cartilage can choose to grow.

Don't increase your max weight too fast. The ligaments and tendons need time to increase before they can support the joints. The recommended limit is a 10% weight increase within eight weeks. This path places cartilage growth before muscle growth.

Stretch often to activate joint health. You can do yoga or Pilates.

Consider car tires when they aren't in alignment. The tires wear out quickly and unevenly. Similarly, when you lift symmetrically, your body will last longer. Lift your weights as straight and steadily as you can.

By lifting in these ways, you may cause pseudo-injuries to the joints. The body then responds by reacting as if it was injured, although it wasn't. When you put pressure on your joints without tearing them, they grow. When the cartilage doesn't tear, the new growth isn't like scar tissue.

While growing cartilage by forming decompression restoration, some pain may be present. New growth can press upon the nerves while the mind signals the bones and cartilage to heal. Certain small pains are part of the process of the mind measuring cartilage thickness.

Keeping physically active increases the rate of cartilage growth. This entire method can help repair spinal discs, cure arthritis, and reverse bone loss due to osteoporosis. It can also help enable the regrowth of hepatocytes, neurons, and cardiac cells.

124

Building the Triangle Wave

You can use a triangle wave for bodybuilding. The triangle frequency is mentioned in chapter 3 of this book.

Triangle wave lifting begins at a lower weight with higher repetitions. Use a progressive load, increasing the weight while lowering the reps. If you choose a one-rep set as your peak, make sure to have somewhat exhausted yourself beforehand so that you aren't actually lifting your maximum weight. After getting through whatever max weight you choose to lift, begin lowering the weight while re-increasing the reps.

Here is a number line signifying the lowering and raising of repetitions in a triangle wave.

– 20-19-18-17-16-15-14-13-11-10-9-8-7-6-5-4-3-2-1-2-3-4-5-6-7-8-9-10-11-13-14-15-16-17-18-19-20 –

When using this exercise system, consider that each number in the line accounts for one minute. Begin in the higher rep range to warm up. Complete two sets in the range from 20 to 15 reps.

Let's say you begin with a 19-rep set before a 15-rep set. There are three numbers between 19 and 15, meaning that three minutes pass between those two sets. You would then wait three more minutes before doing a set of ten reps. If you chose to do a seven-rep set after ten, you would wait two minutes. Do the same thing when relowering the weight. This process keeps the raising and lowering of weight at a steady frequency. When completing the exercise, do two final lifts within the high rep range between 15 and 20.

Imagine that you were going to do sets of ten, eight, and five. That would be ten reps, wait one minute, eight reps, wait two minutes, and then five reps. If it so happened that when you went to do the eight-rep set, you only got seven, you would remain in timing. As long as there are three minutes of rest between sets one and two and sets two and three, then the timing corrects itself.

You don't need to do the same rep numbers when lowering the weight as when you increased. As long as you remain in time, then you remain in the triangle wave.

You can lower the intensity of the lift by observing each number on the line as two minutes instead of one. It doubles the time between sets.

There are also three spiritual rep alignments for lifting. First, avoid doing sets of six reps. Second, avoid doing 16 reps on your sixth set. Third, avoid doing a set of 11 reps right after a set of nine reps.

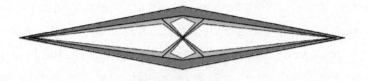

Chapter 8
Supplements

Supplements Considered Mandatory

Vegans need to supplement their nutritional intake with vitamins B12 and D. Forms of supplemental vitamin D are D2 and D3. Vitamin D3 is said to be the best for you. You can also add vitamin K2 if you choose.

Vitamin supplements are recommended only if the ingredients are the essential vitamins along with water and/or food that has passed the guidelines. When choosing vitamins, avoid chemical ingredients.

In the twelfth chapter of the biblical book of Revelation, there is a lady with a garland of twelve stars (or constellations). She is clothed with the sun and has the moon under her feet. The sun signifies vitamin D, and the twelve stars signify B12. The sunshine vitamin is D. The moonlight vitamin is B12.

Imagine living far north in places like Alaska where there isn't much light in the winter. There wouldn't be enough sunshine to provide adequate vitamin D. Clothing yourself with the sun means using a suitable vitamin D supplement. Having the moon under your feet means using a suitable vitamin B12 supplement.

The woman in Revelation chapter 12 is giving birth to a new child. While she is clothed with the sun (her husband), he is clothed with the moon (his wife). He is below her feet because he is helping her give birth. The child wears the sun and the moon and is known as the Lamb. This new child means the vegans. (Revelation 12:1-2) Vegans are considered a new species.

As a peaceful, lamb-like species, vegans must provide reliable sources of vitamins B12 and D without killing or stealing from animals. The biblical book of Revelation states that the city of GOD needed no light from the sun or the moon, and that the Lamb (vegan) would be the light. (Revelation 21:23) That verse means that vegans can obtain vitamin D in the dark or the light, with or without the sun. Therefore, they have the nighttime (moon) below their feet. Vegans don't need direct sunlight to obtain this vitamin.

This Livet revolves around establishing strong bones and cartilage for being active. Calcium for bones works in conjunction with vitamin D, and therefore both are essential. This Livet places the foundation of our house (physical body) on a solid rock where lichen grows. The rain descends, the floods come, and the mighty winds blow and beat against the rocks. Even through hurricanes and tornadoes, the lichen remains solid. (Matthew 7:24-25) A lichen is a group of several plantlike species growing together which produce vegan vitamin D3. (Luke 6:48)

Reading through Revelation chapter 12 reveals that Satan will attempt to war with this new child. While founded on this rock, veganism will survive. Lichen hasn't been considered forbidden at any time. It doesn't grow in the water, nor on manure. Only if we find something better can we stop using this source.

Along with the Livet being founded on the Rock, it also has what is known as the Rod. Vitamin B12 has been made from the fermentation of a rod-shaped bacteria known as Bacillus. B12 is indirectly responsible for raising your blood iron levels through methionine synthesis. B12 is the Rod of Iron vitamin. (Revelation 12:5, 19:15) B12 is a moonlight vitamin because it is involved in making melatonin, which helps control sleep.

Bacteria are not plants or animals; they are mechanisms. This foundation is to remind us that we are granted the use of bacteria, fungus, and algae to make the essential vitamins and enzymes needed for health. Lichen and other forms of D-2 and D-3 are acceptable if needed. They should be produced in sterile environments.

Fermentation happens naturally within the intestines, and although vinegar and alcohol are not recommended, we are allowed to use fermentation to make vitamins that we need, such as B12 and K2. We are allowed to reproduce any type of bacterial process that may also happen naturally within us. We are allowed to perform the procedures needed to survive.

Consider this: if a rat gets inside your home, do you move out or move the rat out? If a virus or deadly bacteria gets into your body, do you decide not to live so that the virus or bacteria can be happy, or do you get rid of it? The Jain key to life, known as Anekantavada, allows us to live rather than to cease to exist. (Ecclesiastes 7:15-16) If you have a vitamin deficiency, you may use suitable supplements to better your health. You are not less righteous when you use acceptable supplements. Your life is important for the beneficial healing of everyone, so take care of it.

Essential Supplements

Here are several suggested supplements for vegan vitamins B12, D2, D3, and K2.

1: Bulk Supplements Pure Methylcobalamin Vitamin B12 Powder – The Ingredient is B12 Powder only and must be measured with a microgram scale. To make a 1 oz dropper bottle of B12, the scale should read .045 grams. The daily recommendation is one dropper per day (not just one drop). Double for a 2 oz bottle.

2: Bio-Alternatives Sublingual B12 (Liquid) – The ingredients are B12 and filtered water.

3: Vegan Ddrops 1000 IU 180 Drops – The ingredients are fractionated coconut oil and vitamin D2.

4: Pure Therapro Rx Full Vitamin D3 + K2 Liquid Drops. The D3 is lichen-sourced and the K2 is made from the geranium flower and/or chickpeas. The other ingredients include coconut and sunflower products. The ingredients have been changed at least once. Check before buying.

5: Givol Vitamin D3 + K2 Liquid Drops. The D3 is lichen-sourced and the K2 is made from the geranium flower and/or chickpeas. The other ingredient is from coconut.

Semi-essential Supplements

Depending on your needs, you may choose to further supplement. This list has some of the safest supplements that vegans can commonly benefit from.

1: B5 Pantothenic Acid (Calcium Pantothenate)
B5 may be low in some vegan diets due to heat from cooking.
This can be found at Bulk Supplements.

2: B6 Pyridoxal-5-Phosphate (P5P)
B6 may be low in some vegan diets due to heat from cooking. P5P is the bioavailable form of B6.
This can be found at Bulk Supplements.

3: B9 Folate
B9 may be low in some vegan diets due to heat from cooking.
This can be found at Bulk Supplements.

4: Potassium Chloride

Potassium may be low in some vegan diets due to heat from cooking.
This can be found at Bulk Supplements.

5: Iodine

Without iodized salt, iodine will likely be low in vegan diets. The recommendation is deep earth iodine. Cedar Bear Pure Nascent Deep Earth Iodine is approved. The other ingredients in this supplement include vegetable glycerin and purified water. Can be found at Amazon.

6: Carnosine

Vegans may be lower in carnosine. This supplement is optional, yet it isn't considered essential.
This can be found at Bulk Supplements.

7: Carnitine – (a combination of the amino acids methionine and lysine)

Vegans may be lower in carnitine. This supplement is optional, yet it isn't considered essential.
This can be found at Bulk Supplements or purebulk.com.

8: Iron – Some vegans may benefit from an iron supplement.

Supplements for Building Cartilage and Bones

This section has a list of some of the very safest vegan cartilage-building and joint support supplements with the least amount of side effects. Check to make sure all products are vegan before buying.

1: **MSM** – Promotes bone and joint health while combating possible vegan sulfur deficiency. Vegan forms can be found at Bulk Supplements and purebulk.com.

2: **D-Glucosamine Hcl Powder** – Promotes bone and joint health and is good for the skin. A vegan form can be found at purebulk.com.

3: **Mythocondro Chondroitin** – Promotes joint growth. This supplement is said to be about 43% more bioavailable than chondroitin from cattle. The vegan form recommended is Doctor's Best Vegan Glucosamine Chondroitin MSM. Currently there is limited availability other than that product.

4: Hyaluronic Acid – Promotes joint health and is good for the skin. A vegan form can be found at purebulk.com.

5: Horsetail (not extract) – Promotes bone, joint, hair, and nail health. Whereas not all silica is bioavailable, the kind in horsetail is. It can be found at Bulk Supplements.

6: Calcium Aspartate – Bioavailable and absorbed well. A vegan form can be found at Bulk Supplements.

7: Calcium BHB Beta-hydroxybutyrate – Absorbed well and helps with recovery. A vegan form can be found at Bulk Supplements.

8: Collagen – There may be some forms of vegan collagen available soon. This supplement can help with bone and joint health.

For maximum bone and cartilage increases, you can make a bone density supplement. Mix 1½ cups calcium aspartate, 1 ¼ cups calcium BHB, and 2 cups horsetail powder. Use 1 to 2 teaspoons daily. This will also help reverse bone loss due to osteoporosis. These measurements could change based on the quality of the supplement. These measurements are based on the current bulksupplements.com products when this book was written.

Muscle Building Supplements

This section has a list of some of the very safest vegan muscle-building supplements with the least amount of side effects.

1: Ceylon Cinnamon – (for maintaining testosterone) Can be found at Amazon.

2: Creatine Monohydrate (Micronized) – Can be found at Bulk Supplements.

3: Shilajit – (for testosterone from fulvic acid and other minerals) The recommendation is to cycle this supplement with three weeks on and one week off. Then four weeks on and two weeks off. Begin again.

4: L-Citrulline DL-Malate – Can be found at Bulk Supplements.

5: Glutamine – Can be found at Bulk Supplements.

Enzymes

Probiotics could possibly change the microbiology of your digestive system permanently. It is always best to allow your body to build its immunity and digestive systems naturally.

Your body makes digestive enzymes. It has been said that using digestive enzyme supplements may cause your body to build dependency on them. If this happens, your body could stop producing enough enzymes on its own. It is best to get your extra digestive enzymes from whole foods.

You should have some of these three digestive enzymes each day.

1: Protease Enzyme – This one breaks down proteins. It is found in pineapple, papaya, and kiwi. It is systemic, meaning that it also enters the bloodstream. Papain is the type of protease in papaya. Though papaya is good, it is one of the most often genetically modified foods. You may want to check the papaya source.

2: Lipase Enzyme – This one breaks down fats. It is found in avocados. The body also produces some.

3: Amylase Enzyme – This one breaks down carbohydrates and starches. It is found in Mangos.

Paragain Supplement

In order for a supplement to wholly function, it must support the entire body. This supplement is intended to do just that. Paragain was designed to target full-body healing all at once.

The twelve herbs chosen are said to have some of the best nutrients for each system or part of the body. According to research, each of these herbs is safe for long-term use. They also follow every rule of the Sculpor's Livet.

The recommendation is to mix an equal number of servings of each of these herbs together. Serving sizes of each one will vary. When the twelve are combined and mixed, measure the total serving size equivalent to all of them together. Begin with half the total serving amount daily. Use five days per week, skipping Wednesdays and Fridays. After three or more months, and if there are no allergic reactions, you can increase to one full serving of the mixture if you choose.

Using pea protein isolate with this supplement could be beneficial. The included amino acids would then be available to help synthesize the nutrients.

Here are the twelve selected herbs.

1: Ajuga Turkest

2: Black Currant

3: Black Pepper

4: Ceylon Cinnamon

5: Chamomile

6: Echinacea

7: Gynostemma (called the herb of immortality)

8: Horsetail

9: Moringa

10: Schisandra

11: Vanilla Bean Powder

12: White Mulberry

This next list has the primary parts of your body. The twelve herbs are mentioned with the areas that they are said to assist.

Blood Cells – Chamomile, Moringa, Vanilla

Circulatory System, Cardiovascular, & Lymphatic – Celyon Cinnamon, Black Pepper, Vanilla

Digestive System – Black Currant, Chamomile, Vanilla

DNA & Telomeres – Celyon Cinnamon, Gynostemma, Moringa

Ears – Schisandra, Horsetail

Excretive System, Kidneys, & Libido – Black Currant, Schisandra

Eyes – Black Currant, Schisandra

Endocrine & Reproductive System – Black Currant, White Mulberry

Hair, Nails, & Bones – Horsetail, Schisandra

Heart – Chamomile, Gynostemma, Vanilla

Immune system – Ajuga Turkest, Black Currant, Moringa, White Mulberry, Horsetail

Joints – Black Pepper, Echinacea, Horsetail

Metabolic System & Liver – Gynostemma, Schisandra

Muscular System – Ajuga Turkest, Schisandra

Nerves & Mind – Ajuga Turkest, Black Pepper, Chamomile, Echinacea, Gynostemma, Moringa, Schisandra, Vanilla, White Mulberry

Nose – Ceylon Cinnamon, Black Pepper

Respiratory System – Lungs & Nose – Black Currant, Black Pepper, Chamomile, Ceylon Cinnamon, Echinacea, Gynostemma, Moringa, White Mulberry

Skin – Schisandra, Vanilla, White Mulberry

Together the twelve chosen herbs form a drink called the Elixir of Immortality, also known as Amrita.

Each of the herbs is chosen using a specific set of guidelines. With more research, the list could change. There are many more herbs that are safe for long-term use and also fit with the guidelines. Eventually this will be absolutely perfected.

Using all twelve herbs together is not recommended during or right after surgery, by those who have medical conditions such as autoimmune or bleeding disorders, or while pregnant or breastfeeding. Some of the herbs are considered unsafe with certain medical conditions. during surgery, or right after surgery. If you choose to use this supplement, you are responsible for learning about any allergic reactions that you may have.

Special Herbs for Ladies

These herbs are said to help with maintaining estrogen in women. They can be added by choice.

1: **Red Clover for Ladies** – Good for Respiratory, Circulatory, Skin, Hair, Nails, Bones, and Endocrine

2: **Chasteberry for Ladies** – Good for Skin and Endocrine

Extra Herbs

These three herbs are supposed to be great for you. They were not included in the twelve because they usually come in root form. If you could supplement these without the roots, then they would be allowed in the Livet.

1: **Astragalus** 'not root' – Good for DNA & Telomeres, Heart, Blood Cells, and Digestive

2: **Shatavari** 'not root' – DNA & Telomeres

3: **Ashwagandha** (is a nightshade) 'not root' – This herb is said to lengthen telomeres. Good for Nerves, Mind, and Endocrine

According to research, the safest three herbs in the list for pregnant women are Ceylon cinnamon, chamomile, and black pepper.

The two herbs that were considered for the supplement yet were considered possibly unsafe by some people were ginkgo biloba and alfalfa powder.

Ginkgo biloba is beneficial to the Nerves, Mind, Respiratory System, Lungs, Nose, Circulatory System, Cardiovascular System, Lymphatic Systems, Blood Cells, Eyes, and Ears.

Alfalfa powder is good for the Immune System, Excretive System, Kidneys, Libido, Metabolic System, Liver, Respiratory System, Lungs, Nose, Digestive System, Skin, Hair, Nails, Bones, Blood Cells, DNA, and Telomeres. One gram daily should be safe.

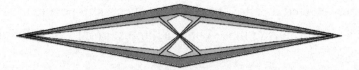

Chapter 9
Spiritual Nutrition Keys

This chapter discusses the spiritual and religious factors of the Livet. The idea is that the Livet can be used to slow and/or reverse aging. This is done by illuminating your nutritional intake.

Here is how it works. Time is thought to slow down as we approach the speed of light. Each righteous and harmless healing path is an expression of light. (Psalm 97:11, 112:4) (Proverbs 4:18, 13:9) (Isaiah 42:6, 58:8) (Ephesians 5:9) Religious foundations and ideas are types of light that are meant to enter our systems. The Livet provides a way to successfully place all of their radiance within us at once. The spiritual notion is that by using this plan, you can increase your frequency towards the vibration of white enlightenment.

Once your nutrition is illuminated, you can then use modern science and technology to go even faster than the speed of light. The thing about science is that while it ages, it continually gets healthier and more accurate. Therefore, science can be seen as if aging in reverse.

Compare this notion to early photos which were on paper and had to be developed. Photos later became ageless and can be transferred digitally. Science gets healthier over time, allowing better products that last longer. This is similar to healing. As we connect the light of righteousness to science, the Livet gets healthier. Once you internally attain the speed of light with the Livet, adding science can propel you faster than the speed of light. Aligning your frequency to light and science helps enable and promote reverse aging.

The Three Spiritual Families

The foods for the Livet were selected by allowing the most successful people in history to offer suggestions. In this definition, most successful refers to those with the largest groups of individuals believing in them.

The path for selecting those who got to offer these suggestions was found in doctrine. Throughout time, many religions have been born. The Bible has a map of how to fit them all together.

In the Bible there was said to be a man named Noah who had three sons. It was thought that the entire world was populated by their descendants. Their names were Shem, Ham, and Japheth. That was long ago.

Years later, a man named Abraham had eight children with three women. Each woman descended from a different son of Noah. Abraham later split gifts between his sons so that the entire world of spirituality would receive them. Together his children would set out to build various religions that promote peacefulness and righteousness. The right to bring these religions together into one was given to his son Isaac. This means that all of Abraham's children were placed in Isaac's hands. (Genesis 25:1-11)

Because there were many types of individuals, numerous religions were designed. Each religion was intended to gather people based on their distinct personality types.

The world became spiritually populated through the gifts of Abraham. This spiritual population is one body, properly known as the body of Jesus Christ. It is the oneness of the spiritual families of Shem, Ham, and Japheth. These religions function together, bringing morality and help to the world. (1 Corinthians 12:27)

Each religion has its own path to veiling and revealing the three families of Noah and Abraham.

These families were veiled in Confucianism as the three aristocratic families called the Huan. The three Confucian families were Ji, Meng, and Shu. All three were to be under the authority of Abraham, whom they called the Duke.

The Ji family is considered the minister over the masses. This signifies Shem as the Christians and Jews. They had the covenant of the Bible, meaning that they are the minister. The Bible was designed with a map to put the families together, which was what Abraham gave Isaac.

The Meng family is the minister of works. This aligns to the builders and merchants of the Biblical Japheth. (Genesis 10:2, 25:1-4) (Ezekiel 27:1-36) The Japheth family is the alternative religions.

The Shu family is the minister of war. This aligns with the Biblical Ham. (Genesis 16:12) The Ham family is the Baha'is and the Muslims. Ham's job was to set up a decoy antichrist and a decoy Babylon. That was how they cloaked Biblical meanings to minister spiritual warfare.

In Taoism, Jesus is called the Son of Heaven. In Taoism the three families are known as the Three Ducal Ministers. Whereas this term was thought to be meant for the emperor of those days, it wasn't about him at all. That was their spiritual veil. The Son of Heaven is Jesus.

Here is a Tao Te Ching verse.

(Tao Te Ching 62:3) "Therefore when the sovereign occupies his place as the Son of Heaven, and he has appointed his three ducal ministers, though (a prince) were to send in a round symbol-of-rank large enough to fill both the hands, and that as the precursor of the team of horses (in the court-yard), such an offering would not be equal to (a lesson of) this Tao, which one might present on his knees."

For various Tao Te Ching translations here and throughout the book, you can visit this link.

https://www.yellowbridge.com/onlinelit/daodejing62.php?characterMode=s

Once these religious families were brought together, a complete nutritional path was opened. In order to find a health-based Livet that would be appropriate for everyone, each of the prominent religious foundations was enabled the opportunity to vote. These votes were brought together as one. Veganism became the main goal.

Family of Shem – Visible Body and the Proton Mind

Shem signifies the visible body that you see. Shem was split into 12 portions known as the 12 sons of Jacob. Shem is known as the Word because they had the foundation of the 'Word of GOD' to put the three families together as one. When the three families come together, they form the body of Jesus. (Ephesians 4:11-16) (Colossians 2:1-9) (1 Corinthians 12:12-31)

Head & Proton Mind

The head of the spiritual body of Jesus is the tribe of Judah, seen in all that they do. They are the Southern Baptist Convention, including African initiated churches. Not all churches in Africa are African initiated. Only the multiple congregations that are non-denominational and have a headquarters with several or more churches are included. The head also contains the mind of Christ, or the proton mind. (2 Colossians 2:18-19)

Legs

The legs of the spiritual body of Jesus are the tribe of Levi. They include the 7th Day Adventist Church and the churches that celebrate their Sabbath on Saturday. In the priesthood body within Levi, the Deacons are the feet, the Pastors are the shins and calves, the Priests are the knees and thighs, and the Bishops are the hips. The living law of Jesus is the cartilage and the synovial fluid throughout the body.

Mouth

The mouth of the spiritual body of Jesus is the tribe of Joseph, having been split into two parts, being Ephraim and Manasseh. They hold the symbol of the Abrahamic blessing. Manasseh is the Oriental Orthodox Church, and Ephraim is the Eastern Orthodox Church. The Orthodox Churches are the symbol of the Abrahamic blessing upon the Mormon church, which is also a part of Joseph.

The entire body controls what the mouth says, and the Word is a combined fellowship of all accepted religions speaking as one. If one church claims that they are the only true church, the spiritual meaning is that they are speaking as the entire body of religions.

Nose

The nose of the spiritual body of Jesus is the tribe of Reuben, which is the Catholic Church.

Ears

The ears of the spiritual body of Jesus are the tribe of Simeon, which is the Presbyterian and Reformed Churches.

Tongue

The tongue of the spiritual body of Jesus is Naphtali, which is the Pentecostal Church.
(James 3:1-5) (Genesis 49:21)

Eyes

The eyes of the spiritual body of Jesus are the tribe Gad, which is the Lutheran Church.

Torso

The torso of the spiritual body of Jesus is the tribe of Issachar, which is the Methodist church.

Chest

The chest of the spiritual body of Jesus is the tribe of Asher which is the Anglican and non-denomination churches brought together.

Hands – Including from the Elbows to the Wrists and the Palms

The hands of the spiritual body of Jesus are the tribe of Zebulun, which includes all Baptist churches other than the Southern Baptist Convention.

Arms – Shoulders to Elbows

The arms of the spiritual body of Jesus are the tribe of Benjamin, which is the Jehovah's Witnesses with the Quakers, Amish, and Anabaptists.

Fingers

The fingers of the spiritual body of Jesus are the tribe of Dan, which are those who call themselves Jews, including the Jews for Jesus Church.

Family of Japheth – Internal Organs

Now that Jesus is visible, where are all His organs and tissue systems? Noah said that Japheth would be in the tents of Shem. (Genesis 9:27) The symbolic meanings of tent are wife and body. The Bible states that Jesus' bride is the church, and the church is the body of Christ. (Ephesians 5:23) (Colossians 1:24) Japheth is primarily internal. This means that Japheth is the organs and systems of the body of Christ. Japheth is known as the Light.

Nervous System

Rastafarianism is the nervous system of the spiritual body of Christ. It is sealed to the tribe of Judah.

Immune System and Bone Marrow

Buddhism is the immune system, including the bone marrow of the spiritual body of Christ. It is sealed to the tribe of Levi.

Excretive System and Kidneys

Joseph is aligned to the excretive system, including the kidneys of the spiritual body of Christ. Shinto is aligned with Manasseh, and Confucianism is aligned with Ephraim. Use the mouth to excrete problems by speaking against things such as lies, hypocrisy, and deceit. It is sealed to the tribe of Joseph.

Endocrine and Upper Respiratory Systems

Cao Dai is the endocrine and upper respiratory systems of the spiritual body of Christ. It is sealed to the tribe of Reuben.

Stomach and Digestive System

Hinduism is the stomach and digestive system of the spiritual body of Christ. In scripture, we eat the Word and drink means listen. (Jeremiah 15:16) (Ezekiel 3:1-2) It is sealed to the tribe of Simeon.

Metabolic System and Liver

Zoroastrianism is the metabolic system and liver of the spiritual body of Christ. Liver symbolically means soul, and the tribe of Naphtali leads the Stewards (Patriarchs). Soul means experience and memory. The Stewards are the primary guides of our soul path. It is sealed to the tribe of Naphtali.

Endocrine System in the Mind and Libido

Cheondoism is the endocrine system and the libido of the body of Christ. It is sealed to the tribe of Gad.

Circulatory, Cardiovascular, and Lymphatic Systems

Tenrikyo is the circulatory, cardiovascular, and lymphatic systems of the spiritual body of Christ. This includes all other non-denominational alternate religions that pass the righteous requirements, such as Unity. Any new religion that passes is automatically sealed here unless they are chosen to be sealed somewhere else. It is sealed to the tribe of Asher.

Lower Respiratory System

Taoism is the lower respiratory system of the spiritual body of Christ. Breathing through your stomach (torso area of the tribe of Issachar) is said to be more efficient. It is sealed to the tribe of Issachar.

Skin

Falun Gong is the skin of the spiritual body of Christ. Skin is held within the hands (the tribe of Zebulun) as when a father holds his child. It is sealed to the tribe of Zebulun.

Muscular System

Sikhism is the muscular system of the spiritual body of Christ. It is sealed to the tribe of Benjamin.

Nails, Hair, and Bones

Jainism is the nails, hair, and bones of the spiritual body of Christ. It is sealed to the tribe of Dan.

Family of Ham – Blood of the Lamb (Revelation 7:14)

The spiritual family of Ham is the life of Jesus H. Christ. The blood passes through all religions.

Red Blood Cells

The Muslims are the red blood cells of the body of Jesus H. Christ.

White Blood Cells

The Baha'is are the white blood cells of the body of Jesus H. Christ.

Seal of the Pouring of Blood

If you have read the explanation on sleeping vs. awakened in Chapter 1 of this book, know that the explanation of sin not existing doesn't mean that you can do anything that you want and still live in the Spirit of GOD. There is a forbidden fruit, and we are warned not to eat from it. You can eat from any tree in GOD's garden except for the tree of the knowledge of good and evil. The doctrinal form of the forbidden fruit is the politicians, military forces, officers, judges, lawyers, prosecutors, prison guards, and psychologists of today (as they currently practice). To eat from them means to read into and believe in their ways. Those who believe in their ways have the Devil's knowledge of that which is good or evil instead of GOD's knowledge of good and evil. The governments that lead the people also refuse GOD's guidance at the same time. Those who choose their ways of leadership also believe that they owe honor to them, and that honor is more important to them than GOD's will. Those who stay with them remain asleep.

In the kingdom, you may think that these offices listed as the doctrinal forbidden fruit were the actual white blood cells of Jesus. They are more like an autoimmune disorder in the blood. Look at this quote from the New King James Bible. When reading it, notice the portion highlighted in red. To better comprehend the context and meaning, you may also read the entirety of the verses.

(Colossians 2:20-23) "Therefore, if you died with Christ from the basic principles of the world, why, as *though* living in the world, do you subject yourselves to regulations— "Do not touch, do not taste, do not handle," which all concern things which perish with the using—according to the commandments and doctrines of men? These things indeed have an appearance of wisdom in self-imposed religion, *false* humility, and neglect of the body, *but are* of no value against the indulgence of the flesh."

144

In the Bible, to eat means to read. We are not supposed to read their doctrines. We are not supposed to touch, taste, or handle their doctrines. They are considered the commandments and doctrines of men, meaning humans. They include guns, bombs, war, and prisons. All self-imposed religions accept them and their ways.

The law is that we have to pour the blood out and not eat (read) the doctrine with them in it. (Genesis 9:4) (Leviticus 3:17) Their blood is a doctrine of honor, force, war, blood money, and murder. By law of GOD, their doctrines must be poured out in scriptures in order for them to be true.

If the officers and leaders of the world are considered good examples in the books that people of the religions have written, then those books are by law to be burned. (Leviticus 6:30) Here is an example. A person of the church always preaches about how Satan and Jesus are just like the redcoats and bluecoats during the war between 1765 and 1783. This person continually preaches that these soldiers are a great historic example of the ways of Jesus. So many churches use stories of war heroes as examples of the ways of Christ. These stories are 100% backwards. Those are stories of the devil's wars. The red and blue coats were fighting over power while they were robbing continents from natives by murder. Jesus only fights spiritual battles.

The job is to teach them to fight the good fight. The good fight is a spiritual war within ourselves. We war with our setbacks to become better individuals. This type of metaphoric war is known as jihad. (Ephesians 6:12) Religious leaders are false if they incorporate soldiers and governmental teachings in their ways.

Since the churches have connected to the governments, they have become corrupt. This is known as drinking and eating the blood of Cain. Those who eat and drink of it are part of the sacrifice. (Ezekiel 39:17-20) Once they get a taste of blood, they, like dogs, begin loving the kill. (Ezekiel 33:25) The churches began saying yes to war, guns, bombs, tanks, fighter jets, and the military. They say fight the Muslims. They also said kill the pagans and destroy the women who play with decks of tarot cards. That is how blind their religion was. They had lost their spirituality. So-called Christians had shirts that said: faith, family, friends, flag, firearms. People also passed digital pictures that said stand for the flag and kneel for the cross, with a picture of a kid pissing on the Muslim name for the LORD. See what a taste of blood does to the entire religion. All these ways and all their books are to be burned according to the law of GOD. Pour the blood out. (Leviticus 7:26-27, 17:10-14, 19:26) (Deuteronomy 12:16, 12:23, 15:23) (1 Samuel 14:33-34)

The religions are not to be associated with war or weapons of war. They are to beat their weapons into plowshares. (Isaiah 2:4) (Micah 4:3)

The blood-pouring riddle means to get rid of the entire doctrine that connects worldly government to religion. The doctrine of the government is considered the blood of Canaan of the house of Cain. This Canaan was called a descendant of Ham, which is why they are so closely associated in the blood metaphor. Canaan is Satan's kingdom. If you don't bring their blood into the holy place, then the doctrine can be eaten (read).

145

(Leviticus 10:18) Clean meat and blood are both offered on the altar of the LORD. The only blood we are allowed to eat and/or drink is the actual blood of Jesus H. Christ, which is the religious family of Ham. (Deuteronomy 12:27) (John 6:53-56) (1 Corinthians 11:27)

The kingdom of heaven is designed using religions from three families. The governmental groups mentioned as the forbidden fruit are not a religion. The ideas that formed them didn't come from spirituality. They are not part of the kingdom of GOD.

The original forbidden fruit was the eating of meat. Eating meat leads to increases in warlike behavior. Eating meat causes war and hunting to become like a sport to the people. (Baruch 3:17) Killing to eat meat leads to murder being a normal behavior throughout society. This then leads to an autoimmune disorder that increases the military mindset of humanity. A military mindset leads to military-based nations. Military-based nations become empires of control, and empires fall.

Eating meat also leads to health problems such as heart disease, pneumonia, diabetes, cancer, stroke, and infections. This next website listed has information on some of the risks of having meat in your diet.

https://nutritionfacts.org/blog/how-animal-proteins-may-trigger-autoimmune-disease/

In the beginning, the rulers of the governments of the earth were the tree of the knowledge of good and evil. The meat was the fruit of the knowledge of good and evil. The meat leads them to the fruits of military empire ways. (Jeremiah 17:10, 32:19) An entire world under the control of military empires dies. This means that eating meat eventually kills the entire Earth, and humanity goes back to the dust as an extinct species.

If you have eaten the forbidden fruit, then you can be cleansed by the blood of the Lamb. The Lamb of GOD signifies veganism. (John 1:29-36) (Revelation 7:10-17, 14:4) The first fruit of the Tree of Life is to be vegan. Adopting a vegan lifestyle helps you rewire the synapse of your mind back into the path of GOD. A vegan world survives because it thinks in beneficial and peaceful ways.

Remember that only GOD would know good and evil, if evil were to even exist. We don't know the difference, and only GOD can show us upon GOD's good will. Stay in the presence of the LORD.

Reproductive System – Birthright of Noah and Abraham

Eyes to Heaven – Astrology is the reproductive system and womb of the spiritual body of Jesus Christ. (John 17:1) (Genesis 22:13) (Isaiah 51:6)

The seed of Abraham was placed into the spiritual womb. The galactic map in Book 7 of this series reveals the spiritual womb. With the keys of heaven, the human species was rewired. That is why the astrology is so different. It is aligned to the Anno Human. It is for the evolved spiritual species.

Together the entire threefold body is the Way of the Love of Jesus H. Christ. His body is symmetric in the path of the Spirit.

Jesus is the King that watches over all these religions. Sometimes He is on earth, and always He is in heaven.

Spiritual Nutrition Guidelines

The optimal nutrition of the third temple Livet is used to take care of the body of Jesus.

Spiritual guides to the Livet were found within the religions. Many avoided foods have been selected based on a spiritual answer. For example, wheat was once thought to have possibly been the forbidden fruit. Long after this notion, celiac sensitivity to wheat has been discovered. Each person may either have found something in the food that wasn't good for them or may have had a vision or revelation regarding the food. Regardless of whether it was due to an instinct, feeling, or a message from a greater being, the founders of these religions were very successful. The Livet incorporates their success within.

By following these guidelines when eating, you can effectively view that the Kingdom is within you. (Luke 17:20-21)

Catholicism
Catholics avoid meat on certain fasting days.

Sikhism
Sikhs follow a lacto-vegetarian diet.

Hinduism

Hindus practice vegetarianism and often veganism.

Mahayana Buddhism

Mahayana Buddhists practice vegetarianism. They don't eat the pungent vegetables such as onions, garlic, chives, green onions, and leeks. They do not use intoxicants.

Seventh-Day Adventists

The 7th Day Adventists practice vegetarianism and often veganism. Alcohol, coffee, tea (with caffeine), and tobacco are avoided. We learn from the Levites that the Law requires us to all be vegetarian as a minimum. We know this because the 7th Day Adventists are the Levites who got that Law directly from GOD. We find proof of this in the book called The Testaments of the Twelve Patriarchs. The table of the LORD was given to those who would be in the temple on the true Sabbath. We are to eat from the LORD's table, which means vegetarian as a minimum requirement.

(Testament of Levi 8:16) "Therefore, every desirable thing in Israel shall be for thee and for thy seed, And ye shall eat everything fair to look upon, And the table of the Lord shall thy seed apportion."

(Testament of Judah 21:5) "dominated by the earthly kingdom. For the angel of the Lord said unto me: The Lord chose him rather than thee, to draw near to Him, and to eat of His table and to offer Him the first-fruits of the choice things of the sons of Israel; but thou shalt be king of Jacob."

From The Apocrypha and Pseudepigrapha of the Old Testament by R. H. Charles, vol. II, Oxford Press

Jainism

Jains practice vegetarianism and veganism and don't eat root foods or tubers nor yeast or honey. They don't eat fungus because fungi don't always naturally grow in a clean place. They don't eat butter, figs, or honey.

One of the goals in Jainism is to not kill plants due to the harvesting of foods. Many Jains eat leafy greens and vegetables such as those harvested by cutting leaves like broccoli and cauliflower. Some Jains don't eat them. Avoiding greens isn't a mandatory rule in Jainism; rather, it is an advanced idea.

Jains wear facemasks to guard themselves from insects, bacteria, dust, and other debris that could be harmful to the lungs. Wearing a mask all the time isn't mandatory, because bacteria is everywhere: where we walk, and even on our skin. Masks are recommended when there are so many insects that they can easily be inhaled.

We are not to make walking and living a burden on ourselves. (Ecclesiastes 12:5) We are not to lay down and wave life goodbye because there are insects or bacteria. We are to live, learn, and avoid harming them the best that we can without allowing them to harness our lives. We don't chain ourselves down. Do not worry about working with bacteria, as they are single-celled mechanisms having been created for purposes of carrying out processes of chemistry. The goal is non-violence, yet we must have the courage to stand and live. Be safe. If we were afraid of harming bacteria, then we wouldn't walk or wash our skin. As we enter veganism, we must supplement with vitamins that require bacterial fermentation. Until we find a better and more advanced way to provide these nutrients, bacteria is an acceptable means for provisions.

Jains boil water to cleanse it from harmful bacteria and viruses. Filtering water is a great idea. Jain regulations also somewhat restrict the use of probiotics.

Taoists

Taoists practice a wide range of dietary rules such as pescatarianism, vegetarianism, or veganism. They don't drink alcohol or eat heavily processed foods like sugar, white flour, fast foods, or foods with preservatives. They don't eat pungent vegetables, including garlic, ginger, and onions. Taoists also avoid eating roots or overly spicy vegetables.

Many Taoist diets today consist of about 50% grains or more. It was said that in the past Taoists didn't eat grains such as rice, corn, and wheat, yet today Taoists do. Some Taoists today don't eat brown rice. Abstaining from these grains has been called Bigu.

The grains avoided in the Livet are actual grains by definition. Grains are seeds from grasses. The Bible states that all flesh is grass, and that the spirit wars against the flesh. (Isaiah 40:6) (Romans 8:1-13) Pseudocereals are similar to grains, yet they are not actual grains. Pseudocereals are simply seeds of a flowering plant. These include amaranth (considered food of the divine), quinoa, kaniwa, and buckwheat. We must find a way to a fullness of complete proteins, and in doing so we must make a path. John the Baptist, also known as Esdras, ate only flowers for a time. Since John was a Levite, he seconds the vote for providing flower seeds as food. (2 Esdras 9:24-26)

They also have five areas of food taste management. Taoists are not to eat foods that are too spicy, too sweet, too bitter, too salty, or too sour. These extremes can reduce digestion and affect the way that the mind reacts to food. Each of these flavors can be eaten in moderation.

Whatever feels good to the five senses often becomes the dietary direction, and that way can be similar to the path of using drugs. (Tao Te Ching 12:1, 63:1) This Livet trains the mind to rewire its synapses so that the body reacts to nutrition instead of flavor. All in all, when the body relies on flavor, it also learns to be dependent on satisfying the senses instead of what is good for you. This creates a domino effect throughout the entire mind, body, soul, and spirit.

Zoroastrianism

The Zoroastrians have claimed vegetarianism would be very important in the last days.

Judaism

With Judaism you will find the exclusion of yeast, melons, cucumbers, leeks, and meat, including fish. These foods are removed because the people complained to GOD about not having them. The nutritional Livet reveals that we don't complain about it. We get what we get, and we don't throw a fit. (Numbers 11:4-5)

Biblical advice is to also avoid salt, for every sacrifice is to be seasoned with salt. We are not a sacrifice. (Mark 9:49) We avoid the use of iodized salt. The foods in the Lived don't provide enough sodium to remain healthy, so we must incorporate sodium. Sea salt is only acceptable in the amount for our optimal health and isn't considered an a mere seasoning.

Avoid cane sugar and flax. Removing flax isn't a requirement, yet it is a possible suggestion unless needed.

Avoid vinegar because it was refused by Jesus at the crucifixion. Jesus was said to have died right after refusing the vinegar, which reminds us that certain vitamins, such as B12, do come from fermentation processes. Don't give up your B12.

Grapes are avoided by Nazarenes. Jews consider those who refuse to prepare grape products forbidden, and the one time that grapes are ever used in this diet is for an ordinance called communion with wine.

Aligned with the story of Jonah, everything from the sea and water, such as seaweed and watercress, was removed. Jonah was thrown overboard a ship and was later found with seaweed (sea vegetables) wrapped around the head. (Jonah 2:5) This Livet has all water plants, including watercress, removed. This helps us single out the type of nutrient-dense foods we are searching for. If there was a water plant worth eating, it may be duckweed for the B12 content.

Daniel of the Book of Daniel was described as vegan. Daniel and his friends would only eat vegetables and none of the king's delicacies. The king of Babylon was condemned for eating meat. He lost his kingdom and

150

went insane, most probably signifying B12 deficiency. He later ate grass and regained his sanity. This could be because B12 was in the grass (possibly wheatgrass). This reminds us that we are allowed to eat grasses, such as wild rice, when needed to survive.

If you were unable to live without B12, bacteria can be used when needed to survive.

Finally, humanity was said to have been cursed with thistles and thorns. When eating the Livet, you eat nothing forbidden, and you don't inherit a curse. The guidance is to remove foods from plants with thorns. (Genesis 3:17-19)

Falun Gong

Falun Gong forbids the killing of animals for food.

Eastern and Oriental Orthodoxy

Eastern and Oriental Orthodox Churches practice vegan fasting without alcohol and olive oil. Some exclude all oils during fasting. The guidance here is to avoid oils on Wednesdays and Fridays in a constant fast.

Rastafarianism

Rastafarians avoid coffee, alcohol, and tobacco. Many of them are vegan. They don't eat food that is genetically modified, artificially flavored or preserved, or chemically altered. Salts and meats are avoided, as well as some or all dairy products. They also cook foods lightly instead of heavily. They do accept sea salt for nutritional requirements.

Mormonism

Mormons avoid coffee and tobacco. Some also avoid sugar, chocolate, meats, cheeses, and certain spices. They do approve wholesome herbs.

Jehovah's Witnesses

Jehovah's Witnesses don't use tobacco.

Muslims

Sufi and Islamic practices include vegetarianism. Muslims avoid coffee, tea, and many other stimulants.

Baha'i

It was recorded that the eldest son of the founder of Baha'i, Abdu'l-Baha, said that fruits and grains will be the foods of the future. Some people identify the meaning of grains as all seeds. In this definition only, fruits and grains would line up directly to the divine gateway of food in Chapter 6 of this book. The Divine Gateway is only found when all religions are connected, and that is the purpose of Baha'i.

Astrology

Pythagoras said that the fava bean resembles the gates of hell. Avoiding fava beans was input as an astrological nutrition guide. Eating pomegranate seeds according to the Greco-Roman story of Pluto/Hades was how Persephone was abducted. Avoiding pomegranates was also input as an astrological guide.

Foods Thought to be Forbidden

There were other foods that have been considered or depicted as forbidden throughout history. Information about these was found on Wikipedia and other sources.

Grape, wheat, banana, Lumia pear lemon, grapefruit, and quince have been thought to be forbidden.

Fig is a meat eater like a Venus flytrap.

Apples were often depicted as forbidden in paintings.

Poppy has been described as gall at least once. Some forms of poppy are used to make opium.

Psychedelic mushrooms were considered the forbidden fruit by some people.

Palm fruit contributed to much rainforest deforestation. The mass deforesting is problematic.

Hemp seeds have some THC in them and are related to marijuana. Hemp seeds were not included because some people are highly sensitive to THC, which can cause inflammation in the joints. This makes the joints feel like there isn't any lubricant in them and causes pain.

Manufactured foods, including canned foods such as vegetables, beans, etc. are avoided.

Genetically modified foods, including yellow squash, zucchini, soybeans, corn, papaya, canola, alfalfa, sugar beets, potatoes, Arctic apples, rice, and pink pineapples, have been the reason for major court battles that have diminished and ruined many innocent farmers. This Livet doesn't destroy, and therefore whether or not genetically modified foods are good or not, we don't choose to participate in destroying farmers. Soy has been said to be the leading genetically modified seed warred over.

Religious Fasting Keys

Continuing to eat from this Livet is considered a constant fasting. We are not required to remove the foods that are associated with every religious fasting. If you were to continually fast in every way that all of these religions offer, then you would not eat at all. For instance, Jains have a fast for each type of food, including water. (Matthew 9:14-15)

While there are numerous religious ways of fasting, if you choose to do a special Jain fasting, taking out leafy green vegetables, including cauliflower, is promoted. This is called Paryushan. It is the most important fast they have because it is done so that the insects get those plants for a while. It is a fast of consideration for others. May GOD bless those who attend this fast.

The Ancient Way of Food

The Taoist Zhuangzi describes a "divine person" who does not eat grains but mysteriously helps them grow. Here is the explanation. The Bible states that the people of the church are the wheat, meaning that they are the grain. (Matthew 13:24-30) (Luke 22:31) We don't need to read from the current translations of the people in these religions. Those translations usually have the blood of Canaan within them as previously explained in this chapter. What a divine person does is mysteriously help the religions (grains) grow.

The ancient Daoist text called the "Writings of the Masters of Huainan" says: "Those who eat meat are brave but cruel. Those who eat Qi have bright spirits and long lives. Those who eat grains are intelligent but die early, Those that do not eat at all are immortal."

Qi and Qi Gong in food form is the nutritional Livet as introduced in this book. Qi is the nutrition standard of each individual religion. Qi Gong is (Livet), the greatest form of Qi, which is a form of spiritual nutrition. Qi Gong is all religious nutritional standards put together as one.

When it says that those who don't eat at all are immortal, it doesn't mean that they don't actually eat. One meaning of not eating is that you are no longer living in this realm. Another meaning of not eating is to not eat the foods that the religions recommend not to eat and/or you practice your fasting. You become immortal by being sealed in heaven through your example of peacefulness and obedience.

Here are the religious fasting rules.

Religious Fasting Days

You can choose to do one or more fast, and each one adds a blessing. If you put these together into one calendar, you can complete the intermittent fasting in a year.

Southern Baptists

They encourage private fasting.

Seventh Day Adventist

They fast when called to do so.

Orthodox

Xerophagy is a level of fasting with all raw vegan vegetables, nuts, and fruits. This is usually reserved for Good Friday. Strict fasting is vegan without oil and alcohol.

They fast on Jan 5th, September 14th, and August 29th.
On August 1st – 15th they practice the same fasting rules as Lent.
They fast beginning the second Monday after Pentecost (June 5th till June 29th during 2023)
Pentecost is 50th day after Easter Sunday.

On March 9th and 26th, and on June 28th they fast from oil and alcohol.
On Good Friday they don't eat at all.

Lent is 40 days ending the Sunday before Easter. Feb 22nd to April 7th during 2023 – During the second week of lent they only eat two meals on Wednesday and Friday.

Mormonism

They fast on the 1st Sunday of each month for 24 hours where they don't eat or drink at all. They can drink water if it is required for health issues. The resources that they save during fasting goes to feed those in need.

Catholicism

Those between the ages of 18 and 59 fast on Ash Wednesday and Good Friday (Feb 22nd and April 7th 2023). During these days they eat one full meal, and two small meals or snacks which together don't make up an entire meal.

They fast on Lent which is the 40 days prior to the Sunday before Easter.

Presbyterianism and Reformed

Fasting is voluntary for them.

Pentecostal

Their fast begins the first Monday after Pentecost (May 29th till June 29th during 2023).
Some begin on the second Monday after Pentecost. Pentecost is 50th day after Easter Sunday.

Lutheran

They encourage fasting without requirements.

Methodist

They encourage private fasting.

Anglicanism

They fast during the Ember days of Wednesday, Friday, and Saturday following December 13th.
They fast on the first day of Lent, on Pentecost, and on September 14th.
They also fast on all Fridays other than those between December 25th and Epiphany January 6th.

Baptist Churches

Encourages private Fasting.

Jehovah's Witnesses, Quakers, Amish, and Anabaptists.

Fasting isn't required by Jehovah's Witnesses.

Amish fast on Epiphany January 6th, Good Friday, and something called Off Sunday which can vary between communities. On February 26th, they don't eat after noon.

Hebrews

For Yom Kippur they fast from food, drink, bathing, intercourse, anointing, and leather shoes.

They also fast on the day after Rosh Hashana, the 10th of Tevet, the day before Purim, the 17th of Tammuz, and "the 9th of Av which is a 25 hour fast". Bathing, intercourse, and anointing were not included in the fasting rules in Chapter 5 of this book because the focus in on food. Leather shoes should always be avoided by vegans because they are not vegan.

Buddhism

For Buddhists, fasting isn't a requirement. They do intermittent fasting where they are not to eat after the noon meal.

Buddhists do one-sessioner's practice and only one meal per day. These rules are important to the Catholic ways of fasting which include one meal per day and two snacks which cannot add up to a complete meal. These Buddhist and Catholic fasting rules were combined by eating meals before noon.

Also, Nyungne consists of two days. On the first day Buddhists don't eat after noon and the second day they do not eat or drink at all. There is no specific day to do so. This means that we can combine this with days such as Yom Kippur, where they fast from drink, and don't eat after noon the day before.

Rastafarianism

They don't have a fast.

Sikhism
Fasting isn't necessary to them.

Hinduism
Once per week on any day they don't eat till afternoon, yet water can be consumed. This fast can be integrated into different fasts.

Zoroastrianism
They don't require fasting, yet they don't eat meat for four days per month on the 2nd, 12th, 14th and 21st.

Jainism
They fast on the 8th and 14th day during each lunar fortnight. The fast includes perfumes, deodorants, bathing, and hats, and they spend time somewhere special meditating and cleansing. Perfumes, deodorants, bathing, and hats were not included in the fasting rules in Chapter 5 of this book because the focus in on food.

During Paryushan they fast from green and leaf foods (meaning leafy greens; kale, collard greens, broccoli, cauliflower, etc. for 8-10 days between August and September.

They also practice eating before sunset.

Taoism
They can fast on days that they choose as special.

Baha'i
Between the ages of 15 and 70, they fast from March 2nd to March 20th. During these days, they fast from food and drink while the sun is up.

Muslim
They fast through month of Ramadan "March 22nd to April 20th 2023. During these days they eat only before and after sunrise.

The fasting plan mentioned in Chapter 5 of this book was set to the year 2023. This was done because the religious fasting dates shift somewhat each year. Instead of you having to recalculate the fasting days repeatedly, the set chart is alright to use if you choose. Anyone who wishes to retune the fasting days to the current year may also do that.

The Livet is the nutrient intake of Omnism. When the religion were put together to manifest the Livet, it became the spiritual OM of nourishment.

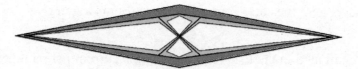

Chapter 10
Scientific Nutrition Keys

This chapter discusses the scientific factors of the Livet. The information provided for the nutritional intake of the Livet came from an estimated thousands of researched websites. The data was compared and sorted to find the answers written in this book. Since the author went through so many different websites to gather material, they are not all mentioned.

Much of the data for the foods was gathered from the site in this link.

https://www.myfooddata.com/

Though the purpose of the list of foods is sure, in the future, as more research is found, the list can be gone through again. The science of the Livet can alter throughout time as more accurate data becomes available.

The Sculptors Livet is based on eating foods that are moderate glycemic-producing. This helps the body build a dependency on complete nutrients instead of sugars. Removing root foods is one of the keys to doing this. The Livet also helps reduce the intake of antinutrients.

This path provides enough methionine to be considered a functional, complete protein intake while still having the possibility of attaining the benefits of a lower methionine consumption if chosen.

In Chapter 4 of this book, there is a section with a list of 84 approved foods. The list of foods had to be reviewed to pass all scientific nutrition guidelines. The foods were then checked for 21 micronutrients. The numbers before the foods in the list signify how many of the 21 micronutrients are at least 10% or more the daily recommended value in one cup of each food. The micronutrients tested for and numbered with the foods are: A Vitamin RAE, B1 Thiamin, B2 Riboflavin, B3 Niacin, B5 Pantothenic Acid, B6 Pyridoxine, B9 Folate, Beta Carotene, C Vitamin, Calcium, Choline, Copper Cu, E Vitamin, Iron Fe, K1 Vitamin, Magnesium, Manganese, Phosphorus, Potassium K, Selenium Se, and Zinc Zn. Iodine and K2 were so minimal that their contents were not listed.

The 84 foods are listed that way because many of the 21 vitamins and minerals function in conjunction with one another. Certain micronutrients, such as vitamin A and beta-carotene, should be consumed together. Calcium, magnesium, and phosphorus should also be eaten together. Iron and vitamin C should be eaten together. The higher numbers help the eater connect more nutrients together at once.

Many foods that are not mentioned in the list are allowed. This current list includes the best-known common foods in stores that most people should have access to. Foods can also be added in the future.

While all foods on the list are considered anti-inflammatory, some foods, such as tomatoes, chia, okra, and peppers, are possibly neutrally inflammatory, meaning that they may have both inflammatory and anti-inflammatory properties.

This Livet is founded upon strengthening the bones to improve cartilage health, thus allowing the eater to remain in motion. If a listed food has greater amounts of calcium, magnesium, phosphorus, selenium, and vitamin K than average, that was mentioned. These specific vitamins and minerals are needed for bone health.

The main micronutrients needed to build bone density are calcium, vitamin D3, iodine, vitamin K, magnesium, manganese, phosphorus, potassium, selenium, and silica. To complete the micronutrients for bone growth, iodine, vitamin D, and K2 supplements are recommended. Some silica can be gained by eating green beans, leafy greens, and nuts. Not all silica is bioavailable, and your body must break it down first. A horsetail supplement is great for adding silica because the orthosilicic acid in horsetail is a bioavailable form. Manganese is also needed for bone density, yet it was not listed with the foods because a great amount is found in many of the foods, especially beans, nuts, and the pseudocereals.

Some vitamins and minerals are affected by heat, freezing, light, or air. According to research, this next list contains the nutrients that are impacted the most.

B-5 pantothenic acid (sensitive to heat and freezing)
B-6 pyridoxine (sensitive to heat and light)
B-9 folate (sensitive to heat)
Vitamin C ascorbic acid (sensitive to heat)
Vitamin E tocopherol (sensitive to air and light)
Potassium (sensitive to heat)

Anti-nutrients Found Within Foods

Along with nutrients, there are also anti-nutrients found in many foods. Most mild so-called plant toxicants also have health benefits with antioxidant values. While the Livet helps you avoid as much of these toxicants as you can, reasonable amounts are acceptable to attain certain benefits. Here is a list of the antinutrients with some helpful ways to avoid them.

Acrylamide

This antinutrient is said to be increased with heat from baking, frying, and roasting. Some of the highest concentrations of acrylamide are in French fries, potato chips, and foods made from grains such as cereals, crackers, and toast. It can also be found in coffee. Roasted nuts have more acrylamide and less phytic acid. If you are going to roast or stir fry, it is best to do so in medium heat, which produces less acrylamide than high heat. Boiling and steaming aren't known to produce acrylamide.

Chaconine

This antinutrient is said to be found in corn, root vegetables, and tubers. Related to solanine, chaconine is avoided through this Livet by eliminating these foods.

Gluten

This antinutrient is said to be found in certain grains. The Livet avoids eating grains with gluten in them.

Isoflavones

This antinutrient is said to be found in soybeans. The Livet reduces isoflavones by keeping soy intake low or eliminating it altogether.

Lectins

It is said that some vegetables have the antinutrients known as lectins. Lectins are considered beneficial to health in certain ways, so removing all of them isn't necessary. Foods with these antinutrients are often considered better for you when steamed or boiled and drained, which helps remove these. Those who eat only raw fruits or only cook seeds should probably avoid foods with lectins a little more than others. The Livet avoids as many lectins as it can while remaining a nutrient-dense food supply.

Oxalic Acid

It is said that some vegetables have the antinutrient oxalic acid. Consider eating fruits and vegetables high in vitamin C moderately yet plentifully. Too much vitamin C can be converted into oxalates. Oxalic acid may help in digestion, so completely removing it isn't necessary. Foods with oxalic acid are often considered better for you when steamed or boiled and drained, which helps remove it. Those who eat only raw fruits or only cook seeds should probably avoid foods with oxalic acid a little more than others. The Livet avoids as much oxalic acid as it can while remaining a nutrient-dense food supply.

Palmitic Acid

This antinutrient is said to be found in certain foods such as dairy and oils. This type of fatty acid has been shown to shorten the length of telomeres. The Livet helps reduce palmitic acid by removing dairy products and by selecting oils with lower concentrations of this substance. Here is a link that reveals research on this subject.

https://www.ncbi.nlm.nih.gov/pmc/articles/PMC6855010/

Phytic Acid

This antinutrient is said to be found in great concentrations within nuts and seeds. Phytic acid restrains the absorption of minerals in the body by inhibiting digestion. For this reason, the Livet promotes cooking seeds. You may remove seeds and/or nuts from your Livet if you choose. Many foods have phytic acid, which does have some health benefits, yet seeds and nuts have a lot. The information provided states that pistachios and hazelnuts have low phytic acid compared to other nuts, and peanuts have low to moderate levels. Soaking and cooking seeds is said to reduce this antinutrient.

Purines

This antinutrient is said to be found in foods such as animal products, processed foods, and beans. Scientific research states that a greater intake of purines contributes to increased levels of uric acid. Increased levels of uric acid can increase complications of arthritis and gout. To reduce purines, the Livet avoids animal products and processed foods and has a selection of lower-purine beans. Some nutritionists believe that plant purines don't affect you as much as animal purines. Plant purines are said not to be as bioavailable, yet we can reduce them even further.

Saponins

This antinutrient has been said to be found in seeds and some vegetables. Licorice root and soy have some of the highest levels of saponins. Levels of this antinutrient are said to be reduced by rinsing and thoroughly cooking seeds and foods that have them. Some small seeds are not easily washed before cooking them. Saponins also have many health benefits, so this Livet allows some to be retained.

Solanine

Some nutritionists recommend that people don't eat solanine. Foods said to have this antinutrient include peppers, blueberries, okra, tomatoes, and other nightshade vegetables. Solanine has also been found to be somewhat beneficial for health in certain ways, so removing 100% of it isn't necessary. Completely avoiding nightshades is an option if you choose. Solanine is said to be reduced when these foods are deep-fried or cooked in hot oil. Those who eat only raw fruits or only cook seeds can avoid foods with solanine if they choose to.

Tannins

This antinutrient is kept at a moderate level with the Livet. Tannins are said to have many health benefits, while some people avoid them.

Trypsin Inhibitors

This antinutrient is said to be found in seeds. The Livet avoids trypsin inhibitors by cooking seeds for long enough periods or by boiling them in water. Cooking trypsin inhibitors deactivates them.

Alternate Food and Supplement Choices

If there were no religious guidelines in choosing the foods, these foods would be some of the best to eat. Next to each of these foods and supplements, there is a reason why it was excluded.

18: **Turmeric/Curcumin** (Root) Would be used daily for joints.

14: **Teff** (Grain)

14: **Garlic** (Root and pungent)

12: **Potatoes** (especially red, white, and purple) (Root)

9: **Wild Rice** (Grain)

8: **Ginger** (Root)

3: **Oranges** (Thorns)

2: **Beets** (Root)

1: **Tangerines** (Thorns)

0: **Olive oil** (Thorns)

Frankincense daily for joints (blood of trees – violence)

Vegan docosahexaenoic acid (DHA bioavailable omega-3) from microalgae daily for joints (aquatic)

Astragalus Root Extract (cycloastragenol & astragaloside for telomeres) (Root)

Muira Puama Bark (for libido, mind, joints, and digestion) (Bark – violence)

Catuaba Bark (for libido, mind, metabolic, and skin) (Bark – violence)

Pine Bark (Thorns and Bark – violence)

Final Notes

1: Your selected foods should increase antioxidant and flavonoid intake.

2: Avoid corn because it is a grain that turns to sugar.

3: If you do eat corn, blue and purple corn have more antioxidants.

4: Avoid white and jasmine rice as they are fillers and not a complete nutrition.

5: The Himalayan Pine Tree isn't thorny. It needs to be researched for edible parts and nutrition benefits.

This Livet is spiritually and scientifically the very best nutrient intake you can have. It can also be scientifically adjusted to make it even better than it is in this book.

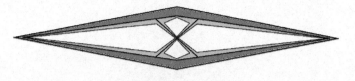

Chapter 11
Final Seals

External Healing

The mind and body are conscious of what you are doing externally. For example, when we plant trees using the Livet, we provide clean oxygen and a healthier environment. Your body becomes more responsive to external increases when you are the one producing them. The external and internal actions then interact with each other.

Carefully selecting fruits and nuts from trees requires trees to be planted. When eating from the 12 fruit trees and tree groups included, the Livet ensures that more are established. Your yearly nutritional intake could require the food from ten or more trees. Eating moringa leaves also provides that trees are planted.

People live in areas of the world with very limited growing seasons. There are different fruits for each month and at different times of the year. Though it is best to gather foods from within your own continent, you can have imported foods from other lands as needed.

It is said that the tree of life bore twelve fruits, each tree yielding its fruit every month. (Revelation 22:2) When everything was calculated, the Livet produced a path with twelve tree types. With these twelve types of trees, fruit is yielded each month. Here are the twelve tree types.

1: Avocados – Yields all year
2: Coconut – Yields from January to December
3: Guava – Yields from February to April and October to December
4: Mulberries – Yields from July to August
5: Papaya – Yields all year
6: Hazelnut – Yields from August to October
7: Macadamia – Yields from March to September

8: Soapberry Fruits

8: Lychee – Yields from May to June

8: Rambutan – Yields from May to July

9: Ericales Fruits

9: Persimmon – Yields from August to December

9: Brazil Nut – Yields from December to March

10: Juglandaceae Fruits

10: Walnut – Yields from September to November

10: Pecan – Yields from September to November

11: Anacardiaceae Fruits

11: Mango – Yields from May to October

11: Pistachio – Yields from August to September

11: Cashew – Yields from March to May

11: Spondias Mombin – Yields from July to September.

12: Prunus Fruits

12: Cherries – Yields from April to July

12: Apricots – Yields from May to July

12: Peaches – Yields from May to October

12: Plums – Yields from May to October

12: Prunes – Yields from May to October, typically August

12: Pears – Yields from August to April

12: Almond – Yields from August to September

Being Vegan for Moral Reasons

It has been estimated that the average person in North America produces about 890,000 pounds of carbon dioxide in a lifetime. That is an average of 445 tons of carbon dioxide pollution per person. We can reduce this by an estimated 73% by being vegan. Your projected average carbon dioxide production per person would be 120.15 tons in a lifetime if you were vegan.

This carbon that humans produce is responsible for much of the atmospheric problems on earth. We, as people, should plant trees to remove our carbon footprint for the fuels we use in everything we do. Consider that the average tree is said to remove about 7 tons of carbon dioxide from the atmosphere. The average vegan would need to plant about 17 trees in a lifetime to remain nonpolluting. If you remained a meat eater, you would need to plant about 64 trees in a lifetime to remain nonpolluting.

To offset the carbon footprint, we must also plant trees for the home we live in. When we emit carbon and use trees, it doubles the offset needed per person. It was estimated that building an average home uses 22 to 44 trees per 2,600 square feet. Consider that you use 33 trees per 2,600 square feet for a wooden house. There are, on average, 2 people per residence responsible for this if married. Even if the people rent a home or apartment instead of owning, they are still using the trees. This would place the average vegan safe by planting 50 trees.

Trees are not only cut for lumber. Trees are also cleared and used for building businesses, schools, and so on. Trees are cleared to build roads and to mine the resources we use. Each person isn't only increasing carbon; they also reduce the amount of carbon that the Earth can cleanse. Because of this, that average of 445 tons of carbon dioxide pollution per person in a lifetime can double. This is based on the reduction of carbon-absorbing trees that each one of us is responsible for removing.

It would be safe to say that a vegan should plant about 100 trees in a lifetime. If you cannot find a place to plant trees safely, you can use donation sites such as One Tree Planted. These sites help reforest. It is also important to know that the successful survival rate of each tree planted could be as low as 50%. Because of this, it is a good idea to plant 200 trees in a lifetime.

One more thing about being conscious is being selfless. We, as people, got in this pollutive position by being overly selfish.

People building too many homes and wasting resources has become a global epidemic. On the North American continent alone, between the years 2000 and 2022, the rate of vacant homes was said to have fluctuated somewhere between 14 and 19 million. During those years, the homelessness rate in North America was reported to be somewhere between 550,000 and 700,000 people. Why would there be that many empty homes in the first place when there were many fewer homeless people?

The answer is an epidemic of selfishness. Some families, as few as two people, live in five- to ten-thousand-square-foot homes. It isn't about them being wealthy or not; it is about the resources they carelessly took from others so that they could have what they wanted.

Next we must consider that though the vacant homes were up to 19 million, that probably doesn't include homes owned by people who have more than one. Some people may not report a vacancy where they have two or more homes. Some people have five or more homes. It may not include apartments and condos. Many condos are owned by people and are only visited once in a while. Then we have hotels and timeshares. Those 19 million empty homes are dwarfed by the reality of how many shelters the continent has that are able to house people. Then add in empty businesses.

There are many businesses that are built where lots of land had to be cleared of trees, while there was lots of land nearby without trees already. There wasn't regard for the environment and resources. Each person was just trying to make as much money as they could.

Who decided that our forests can be cut down carelessly? Who sectioned those resources off as theirs? When you see that the law is designed to uphold that type of behavior, then you begin to wake up. Claiming that as long as it is legal, then it isn't wrong, is an excuse and a cover.

Money and profit have controlled people while the earth was selfishly destroyed. People attempted to get above the market. Banks own much or most of those empty homes and buildings. And most empty homes were built for selfish reasons. There are rental homes being built, while there are millions of empty homes available. Each rental drives up the cost of materials, and the owner rents out the home so that the renter pays for the cost of buying it for them. Building rentals is a selfish money scheme. Building rentals destroys the earth. The people are not only using the resources; they are making it harder for the homeless to afford a home. The people ran up the cost of materials while building more homes for themselves and caused others to pay for those extra homes for them.

Who originally decided not to work together?

Anyone with the idea that money is the true path of wealth should keep walking until they wake up. Conscious people are above the money schemes of the world. Even though a conscious being may not be as wealthy as someone willing to cheat to get the upper hand, they are better for the environment and for everyone. Conscious people make decisions based on selfless ideas.

Now, because of the inherent selfishness of people, vegans would be safe to plant 300 trees instead of the 200 that they should plant for their own usage. Vegans should know not to be selfish. Because of this, they can do more than their part. They should plant an extra 100 trees for the trees that others used before them. They have a chance to be selfless and do more than the bare minimum. It would be good if each vegan planted 300 trees in a lifetime. Therefore, they are not only holding down the problem for themselves; they are also pushing back upon the problem for everyone.

There are many more reasons to be vegan, such as the meat industry being the world's greatest water polluter. Here are two sites that explain this fact a little.

https://www.animalagricultureclimatechange.org/report-meat-industry-worlds-biggest-water-polluters/

https://www.nationalgeographic.com/science/article/burger-water-shortages-colorado-river-western-us

Being vegan is a fundamental moral. When you learn not to steal from others and not to kill, you will find that this includes killing and stealing from animals. It is a moral decision.

Internal Healing

The mind has types of consciousness other than that which scientists are currently aware of. The subconscious mind is the mind's own conscious mind of its own. It is aware of what you think and do. Your mind, body, and spirit know in detail what you are eating.

Adapting the spiritual non-kill eating path of the Livet allows the mind and body to recognize that a non-kill system is being ingested. The mind is aware of the nutrient base of combinations within your body. The mind and body then learn the non-kill path that they have chosen to ingest and begin to reflect the same path in the way they heal. Within the Livet, the non-kill system is brought to the best nutritional value available for its day, based on scientific research.

Being Vegan for Personal Health Reasons

Planting trees can extend your life through global systemic unification. A study from Tel Aviv University revealed that high-pressure oxygen can help reverse aging greatly by lengthening telomeres. In a collateral way, we are pressured to increase the oxygen on the planet by planting trees.

You can read about this abstract view on this website.

https://medicalxpress.com/news/2020-11-hyperbaric-oxygen-treatments-reverse-aging.html

Telomeres are used in the reproduction of cells. Being vegan can extend the length of your telomeres, whereas eating processed meat and fish can shorten them, causing an estimated 6 to 14 years of aging. This information can be read at this site.

https://agelessinvesting.com/how-to-lengthen-telomeres/

Other diets, such as being vegetarian and pescatarian, are effective first steps towards veganism. The goal is to learn that the animals are like children or babies. We should not steal from them. It isn't nice to steal their milk or their honey. We would just be big, mean bullies. The fact that people take all that they can from the animals is a direct reflection of their inherent selfish ways. Selfish ways directly and indirectly reflect manifested realities of consciousness and extend into all surroundings.

Being selfless can do the opposite.

Veganism is better for your health. Veganism reduces cholesterol and heart problems.

There are many other things that veganism does to help the environment and your health. If you are truly interested in being a better person for yourself and for everyone, you can watch this documentary called The Game Changers from 2018. It can be found on Netflix and YouTube.

https://youtu.be/YbfXtcaJ7AU

Being conscious includes being willing to look directly at truth and to want to do what is correct for you and for everyone. It means having the spiritual synapse in your mind to be able to see the facts and acknowledge and use them. Being an authentic conscious being begins with veganism. Do you have your seal of authenticity? Are you willing to be better for everyone?

The Meaning of Bigu

The claim is that practicing Bigu starves the three worms that live within your intestines. These worms were said to hasten death so that they can feed on your decay. Bigu was prophetic direction from GOD. Isaac's son Jacob is known as a worm. (Isaiah 41:14)

Those three worms represent the religious families of Shem, Ham, and Japheth. These families have not been awakened. In their current state of not getting along with one another, they hasten the death of Earth, and therefore all people. Here is one example of how they do this. Christians were asked why they don't plant trees. Their response included that the Bible says the trees would be burned up anyhow. (Revelation 8:7) They didn't see that the prophecy was about how their neglectful behavior would cause the problem.

These three families formed many religions that often individually only believed in themselves. Since they rely on only believing in themselves, to arouse them could cause great anguish as they are blind to one another. Many of them have even hated the notion that GOD loves them all. They resemble earthworms which have no eyes.

The earthworms do fertilize the tree of life and are delicate. The religious attendants have not been able to handle the truth. They will eventually receive their eyes. Yet for now they remain in a cocoon state waiting for a spiritual baptism.

Bigu mentions not eating grains. It means not to eat (read) the religious translations of the leaders of the religions. (Matthew 13:24-30) (Luke 22:31) The Bigu prophecy is that humanity will live longer if we don't read into religious leaders' translations of what the scriptures mean. This is because many of them call each other Satan and ridicule one another as if they were the only one. They then hasten death by joining to the governing military states. They grab the power of the officers to fight with one another. Those who grab hold of the officers to justify their ways become one with Satan.

Waking the Eagle

If you look ahead, you'll see the eagle. If you look back, you will see the Lion. Again, if you look back, you will see the Eagle. If you look ahead, you will see the Lion.

The Eagle should signify Abraham's son Isaac connected to the Administration of Angels through Levi. Yet for a long time now it has signified the kingdom of Edom. The eagle eats the worm.

Waking the eagle primarily focuses on the biblical writings of Daniel chapter 7, Revelation chapter 12, and Second Esdras chapters 11 through 14. This part of the book will explain what the beasts in those chapters represent. Reading those scriptures first will help you comprehend the next part of this book.

Evolution of the Religious Beast

Through the books in this series, you can watch the evolution of the beast. The beast is often referred to as the antichrist. Ironically, the Beast is Jesus. He begins as the golden calf that Aaron made. Here we find him in a book of Moses. (Exodus 32:1-35)

Barnabas also spoke about Him.

(Barnabas 8:2) "Understand ye how in all plainness it is spoken unto you; the calf is Jesus, the men that offer it, being sinners, are they that offered Him for the slaughter. After this it is no more men (who offer); the glory is no more for sinners."

The golden calf was a religious idea. It seemed so innocent that it wouldn't harm anyone. Those of the churches who offered it were also they who were slaughtering Jesus. Yes, those who called themselves Christians were those who were killing Jesus. This happened because they had no understanding that Jesus was the idea of anti-war, veganism, and included a foundation of all religions. Those so-called Christians were not the real translators of the Bible's meaning. They were handed a religious code, and whatever their heart already desired was what they did with it.

Jesus was once a harmless idea. The concept of Jesus then grew into an excuse to not do what GOD says and a reason to fight against other people and their religions. We will now examine the prophecy of how Jesus became a war beast.

In this explanation, the body of Jesus is the churches and other religions.

As He grew, that golden calf (Jesus) evolved into a lion. (Daniel 7:2-4) The Christians had the wings of the Word of GOD by which they could excuse anything that they chose to do. They justified eating all the meat that they wanted, even the swine that they were told not to. When they ate meat, their spiritual wings were plucked. This is known as eating the red stew of Jacob. There was red meat in the lentils that Jacob fed his brother. (Genesis 25:29-34)

Christians wanted others to agree with them. They began hunting people to teach them their ways. They were given the heart of a carnal man. Christians decided that if people wouldn't do what they said, then they would have to take control by force.

Governing officials saw that this new religion was a means for gaining power. The government fought against the Christians and became their head. The lion evolved into a bear and became a symbolic woman. (Daniel 7:5) (Isaiah 47:5-9) Christians began eating the fleshy ways of the governments. The officials of the lands became their masters. There were three ribs in their mouth, known as the judicial, legislative, and executive administrations. These three ribs that they had eaten were the forbidden fruits of the nations. The people became raised up on one side. Being raised up means that instead of them administering eye to eye, they practiced domination. Each person felt that they had to be in power over the other. Christianity had become a bear of military power. They were also eating themselves.

Similar to Adam and Eve, once they had eaten from the forbidden fruit, shame and blame became the Christian path. The bear began shrouding itself within a shame-based system. They now used force and humiliation to control the people. Christians started hiding like a leopard. (Daniel 7:6) A leopard, like a leper, climbs to the highest point that it is able so that it can withhold its prey from others. The Christians would hide their prey in shame while devouring them. They were covering their lies.

The leopard had four wings. These four wings were the four groups of religion. The Jews and Christians, being one wing, were the family house of Shem. The Muslims and Baha'is, being one wing, were the family house of Ham. The family of Japheth was the alternate religions. Japheth was split into two houses at this point: Oriental religions and the others remaining. Each of these houses had their own head of government because the nation's leaders presided over them all. None of these four heads of the leopard followed GOD, yet they had dominion over the people.

The beast needed more power as the nations began gathering together. The Leopard became an Iron Dragon. (Daniel 4:7) (Revelation 12:3) The nation of Israel had been split apart long before all this happened. Ten tribes joined themselves to the nations while the other two remained with GOD for a time. The ten tribes became the ten horns of the beast, and they began using the nations to help wage war against other people and religions. This process didn't begin after 34 A.D.; it began about 1,000 B.C. during the days of Solomon. They were being watched the entire time.

During about three millennia, the calf became a lion, which became a bear, which became a leopard, which became a dragon. (Daniel 4:1-7) (Revelation 13:1-2) The entire religious system was now under the war machine. The religions had handed their spiritual authority to the nations. They were all warlike and aggressive. Government officers, legal workers, and politicians were the guides in the religious masses instead of GOD. Each religion was used like a puppet to manipulate a certain amount of control.

The two houses of Japheth had to merge. To do this, Buddhism was sent from Indian lands into the Oriental lands. There in Eastern Asia, Buddhism became infused with the Orient religions. The four heads of the leopard became three when two of them came together. To get the Orients to accept Buddhism, they entered their lands with a religion that refrained from having GOD as a subject. They basically pretended that they didn't believe in GOD.

All twelve tribes of Israel, and all three houses of Shem, Ham, and Japheth, had gone under the nations. The dragon had now become an eagle. The eagle had three heads and twelve wings. Its wings spread over the entire world. The voices (winds) of the religious leaders spoke (blew) in every direction. They sought global domination and the removal of GOD's authority.

This eagle was a beast, and it was also the Son of GOD. This is revealed by comparing chapter 13 in both books of Revelation and Second Esdras. (2 Esdras 11:1-2, 12:11, 13:1-52) (Matthew 26:64)

The religions had become beastly, and their ways were used to fight against the LORD. As a beast, they had symbolically evolved from an innocent calf into an eagle. Religion had become a treacherous predator. Religious attendants looked down upon those who weren't in their own group with an eagle's predatory eye.

The Eagle Fights Itself

The beast is mentioned as coming out of the sea in the books of Revelation and Second Esdras. The son of GOD is also said to be coming out of the sea in the Book of Second Esdras. This is because the entire body of religions is the son of GOD. As a beast of the nations, religions have been on the left hand of power. They had become slayers and needed to be baptized.

Here are some quotes revealing this.

(Revelation 13:2) "Then I stood on the sand of the sea. And I saw a beast rising up out of the sea, having seven heads and ten horns, and on his horns ten crowns, and on his heads a blasphemous name. Now the beast which I saw was like a leopard, his feet were like *the feet of* a bear, and his mouth like the mouth of a lion. The dragon gave him his power, his throne, and great authority."

(2 Esdras 11:1) "The second night I had a dream. I saw an eagle coming up out of the sea. It had twelve wings and three heads."

(2 Esdras 13:32) "When that happens, the signs I told you about earlier will take place, and then I will reveal my son, whom you saw as a man coming out of the sea.

Religions have gone under the governments by which they all died. Non-spiritual guides have been in command of them. The entire eagle needs to be baptized so that it can return to GOD. A baptism is often considered a death and rebirth process. This is one of the meanings of the Hindu rebirth cycle. (2 Corinthians 5:17) (Ephesians 4:22-24)

While governing officials were in charge of the religions, they taught them to fight with each other. They were learning from the type of people who live to fight for power. Without war they have no honor.

The eagle is said to have three heads and twelve wings. The description of the eagle in Second Esdras reveals its hostility towards itself, eating its own wings and heads.

The twelve wings of the eagle are the twelve tribal sections of each of the three families of Noah and Abraham. Each family has twelve, yet all three sets are meshed together. This means that there are really 36 wings, yet only twelve are viewed.

The three families, signified by the three heads of the eagle, were those who supposedly inherited the Earth in Abraham. They ruled with cruelty, upholding the laws and ways of the peoples. Each family of Shem, Ham, and Japheth are a head, and they were asleep while the wings of the body did whatever they wanted. The heads worked together slyly while agreeing to oppress the people for increased power. Yet when the time came to get along, each head fought and ate one another. The entire eagle's body destroyed itself and burst into flames. This behavior was learned by being under the nations.

The unbaptized eagle signifies the world under the oppressive power of the old age. The old age is known as the age of Edom. When it is baptized, the eagle becomes GOD's child with a new Law. The power is to be given back to Isaac, who then places that power in the hands of GOD. (2 Esdras 3:15-16, 6:8-10)

The religions were not taught to get along with one another and live peacefully under the previous age. (2 Esdras 6:7-10) The newly baptized eagle unifies the people and teaches them to get along.

Let's view what this eagle did and what happened to it.

The eagle flew into the air and became ruler of the whole earth and all the people. The religions were military-minded instead of spiritually minded. Cain's spirit had become the one in power within them. No one could oppose the warlike nature of the nations because even the religions sustained their wars. (2 Esdras 11:5-6) (Ephesians 2:2) With government officials in the leadership positions of the religions, they were battle-oriented like the nations. They were all dead to GOD.

The eagle's power is in its claws. With its power, the eagle commanded the wings (religions) not to listen to any truth from anyone called by GOD. This was easily accomplished by them having those who weren't with GOD in charge of the religions. People who serve the nation have been in charge of the religions, and they are enlisted to stand for the nation instead of listen to GOD. The eagle's heads and masters were the nations. It is simple. If a military officer is in charge of a church, then the officer waits for the nation to tell him which way to go. When someone who is called by GOD enters, that person is alien to the church. Men from GOD are considered alien because GOD's direction is to keep all the nations' affairs completely out of the religions. When each religion was inspected, the nations' affairs were nearly all they were attending to.

Using the technique of having the nation's leaders in charge of the denominations, the eagle commands the religions not to all wake up to the truth at the same time. If the religions all woke up at the same time, then they would end the wars, which the government needs to secure authority and honor. Only one religion is allowed to wake up at a time so that the others can fight it.

The book of Second Esdras mentions four wings that rose up to seize power.

Each of these four wings had something that GOD had given them. These wings were the 7th Day Adventists, the Jehovah's Witnesses, the Mormon Church, and the Catholic Church. The 7th Day Adventists have the dietary laws of the kingdom and the correct Sabbath from GOD. The Jehovah's Witnesses have the idea to put the name of the LORD back in the Bible. The Mormons have a large piece of the priesthood that is needed for all of the churches to function together. The Catholics have the idea that all religions can communicate with GOD. The Catholic Church's idea has been under heavy scrutiny. (2 Esdras 11:24-31)

There were eight rival wings on the eagle. Each time one wing (religion) attempted to rise up and do what GOD wanted, the other religions would cling to the government and shoot them down.

One of these rivals rose up to govern the entire world. This is a symbol of the Catholic Church using the Roman Empire long ago. It has long been thought that the Roman Empire was the antichrist. You can see evidence of the Roman Empire living within the nations. The government of the North American continent has what is called a White House. This house is the house of the nation's president. Roman buildings were designed like the Edomite Temple of Mount Seir, known as Al Khazneh Petra Jordan. The White House is also designed in that same specific way. It looks like a Roman or Edomite temple. The government of North America is said to have the world's most powerful military. Their military has been all over in other people's lands like the Roman Empire was. Any church that supports them has bloodshed on their hands. Those who are joined to them are part of the antichrist system.

The Book of Esdras states that the iron beast in Daniel chapter 7 is also the eagle. Here we must review the horns on the iron beast. The horns align to the leaders of the wings. In the book of Daniel, there is a little horn coming up among the others. The little horn caused three of the first horns to be plucked out by the roots. In the little horn were eyes like the eyes of a man and a mouth speaking pompous words. (Daniel 7:7-8) That little horn is the Mormon Church. The three horns that Joseph Smith plucked were the Baptists, Presbyterians, and Methodists. We can see the three churches that he pointed out as false in the Joseph Smith History writings. (Joseph Smith History 1:9)

The pompous words that he spoke included several things. The worst thing that Joseph did was that he indoctrinated the church into the government, saying that the church should go to the leaders of the nation for answers and/or permissions. He indoctrinated himself into the Devil. GOD's regulations are against doing that. There are many biblical verses that are very clear about not joining the nations. The LORD commanded that the religions are not to join any nation in any of their ways. (Joshua 23:11-13, 24:14-15) (1 Timothy 2:5) (Matthew 10:16) (1 Corinthians 11:3)

Here are some examples of how the Mormon Church connects to the government instead of GOD.

1: The church has promoted the buying of war bonds during wars. They support the war efforts, which are blasphemous to GOD. The LORD has never supported a war effort or military soldiers in all of history. (John 18:36) War is carnal, and GOD doesn't have anything to do with it. All of the Bible's wars were fought symbolically and spiritually. GOD never commanded anyone to kill another. Biblical kills are metaphoric and mean spiritual conversions. (2 Samuel 14:14)

2: The church claimed sobriety, which is good for the people. They wouldn't allow those who used marijuana into the temple because it was a drug and it was illegal. Once marijuana was made legal, the church allowed people to enter the temple while on marijuana. The government decided who was allowed in the temple based on national and local laws.

3: The church won't baptize people until they are off probation and done with criminal charges. The courts and their processes are some of the most deceptive things on the planet. When criminal charges are filed by or with the nations, that has nothing to do with GOD. The church allows the courts to decide who gets to be baptized. They teach their doctrines as the commandments of men.

(Matthew 15:8-9) (Titus 1:16) GOD doesn't guide them; the government does. Their doctrine was sealed to the North American constitution and laws, which means that their book was a stillborn child unless otherwise unveiled. Their book must have another meaning or it is from Satan.

4: Those who want to be sealed to their spouses and children in the Mormon temples must have a temple recommend. Sealing in the temple is said to be eternal in heaven. The church holds back temple recommends from those who owe child support. Again, this is allowing the courts to be in charge of heavenly ordinances. When parents split, the rampant deceit that takes place in court battles of custody and support is no part of GOD's ways. One's ability to give money is not to be a part of deciding a heavenly ordinance.

5: The hierarchy of the Mormon church is designed to cut GOD off. The church was built with an order from least to most authority. The leader often works or worked for the government. It is mandatory that church attendants believe and/or practice that the leader is the only connection on Earth to GOD. They must uphold their president's decisions and guidance in all things. That church president is following the guidance of the presidents and leaders of the nations. The Mormon church does whatever the nations say. The nation in North America, for example, practices separation of church and state. The nation denies GOD's authority. If a president is an atheist and/or denies GOD's authority, that president is still in charge of the Mormon president. If you allow a person who is denying GOD to be in charge of you, then GOD isn't the one in charge of you. The church is designed to get you to bow to their leader so that he can cut GOD off of you. That leader then becomes the god of those in the church. They have no god other than the church president, who then bows to the president of the nation. The dual presidents are a design to remove GOD's will. It is a setup.

(Matthew 15:8) "'These people draw near to Me with their mouth, And honor Me with *their* lips, But their heart is far from Me. And in vain they worship Me, Teaching *as* doctrines the commandments of men.' '""

6: The church is indoctrinated to throw out GOD's laws and replace them with the laws of the nations. They have a strong belief, according to their scripture, that says to uphold the law of the land. This is why they follow the nation instead of GOD. When they uphold the law of the nations, they get under the nations and hold them up. This is why the book of Revelation says that the beast carries the harlot. The nation is called the harlot because it is unfaithful to GOD. When the church carries her, the nations, they become like beasts on their way to perdition. (Revelation 17:1-8) That is the way of Cain.

The law of the land actually means that if you cut a tree, then plant a tree. If you make a mess, clean it up. It is very simple. When you use resources, recycle them. Now uphold the real law of the land.

Twin Eagles

Although each wing represents a different religion, they can all be viewed within a seal. The twelve wings align to two groups that merged together. One is a religion, and the other is a nation to which they bowed. They have different timelines that graph together. (Matthew 24:28)

This next explanation is an abridgment as if the wings and/or horns of the beast are the leaders of the Mormon Church. The Mormon Church has been identified as the beast in Revelation chapter 17. In this seal, all the wings were symbolically set within them.

How did this happen?

About 3,000 years ago, ten tribes of Israel separated from Judah during the revolt after Solomon. The ten tribes went with Jeroboam of the half tribe of Ephraim and remained within him spiritually. (1 Kings 12:16-19) Those ten tribes fought with the remaining two tribes for centuries until they were all together displaced. Due to this fact, there is a mirror of all twelve wings being within the family of Jeroboam. This seal is to help identify the house of the beast.

Here are the eagle's wings in the Mormon Church.

The first president of the Mormon church was the first wing. He got tricked by the government and was set up to be killed.

The 2nd president of the Mormon church was the second wing. He joined the government and worked for them after they helped kill the first president of the church. That is how fast the church lost the LORD. The next wing had risen up and governed for a long time. When the rule of the second wing (president) was coming to an end, it was about to vanish. That is when a voice told the second wing that none would rule as long as that one. (2 Esdras 11:13-17) This happened when the Mormon Church almost saw war against the nation during 1857 and 1858.

The 3rd president of the Mormon church also worked for the government. The Mormon church is the family and direct practicing descendant of Jeroboam. They practice the same way of connecting the church to the government as the Herodians did with the Romans, which led to the crucifixion of Jesus around AD 34. (Matthew 15:9)

The early church had joined the government that had overseen the murder of Jesus.

First, the twelve wings are mirrored within the twelve presidents of the Mormon Church. The second wing (president of the church) was in office the longest. As prophesied, the second president (wing) of the Mormon Church ruled longer than the others. The year that the 12th president of the church was ordained by the people was 1973. That president supported the World War II efforts by encouraging the church members to buy war bonds to support the war. That is a blasphemy to all spirituality and to GOD. The government was in the church controlling their wills. Their revelations and wills came from the spirit of the government.

That is the first seal of the eagle. Here is the second.

The second group of the twelve wings is the presidents of the North American government. The North American presidents begin their alignment with the overlapping of the 35th and 36th presidents. The 36th president symbolically ruled the longest based on the fact that he reigned in honor of another person who had been killed. This means that the word of his purpose lasted the longest. The 2nd wing of the nations, the 36th president, passed away during the year of 1973. The year of 1973 aligns these two sets of 12 wings.

The mirror is that both of the first presidents of each group were killed. And in each one, the second wing ruled the longest. Because their rule time is metaphoric, based on the honor of another, none other would ever rule as long as them.

These two eagles are lovers. They are called the beast and the harlot. The church bows to the nation and does their will. By doing their will, the church carries the nation. This is depicted in Revelation chapter 17, where the beast carries the harlot. Nearly all churches did this, yet the Mormon Church directly indoctrinated themselves to do it. Upholding the nation and their military is a direct denial of the Holy Ghost.

The nation's leaders and officers are known in the Bible by the name Baals. They are considered Canaanite gods. A king named Ahab had introduced Baal worship to Israel, which has been considered the worst thing that ever happened to them. When inspecting the Mormon Church, they were celebrating veterans' day. They were publicly honoring soldiers and venerating them. Even their church president was an army veteran.

What they were doing is called practicing Baal worship. It teaches the children that using guns to solve problems is honorable. That isn't even allowed to be a part of the church. As much as the people are unable to understand that the military is Satanic, it doesn't change the fact that it is. Joseph Smith went in the direct way of Ahab. The church denied the Holy Ghost by joining them. This is because by doing so they supported and upheld many murders. (Lamentations 4:19)

Churches are not even allowed to touch warfare. They are commanded to keep themselves clean of all worldly governmental affairs. (James 1:27)

Wings Rise to Govern

Though all of the wings can be seen in the mirror of the Mormon Church, that is only for revealing why the eagle was killing itself. The seal is meant to expose why the religions could not get along with one another. The reason was because they were acting like the nations. They each claimed to be GOD's true religion while denying GOD's ways. (Psalm 2:1) (Acts 4:24-26)

Now we will view the wings from the assessment of the house of Japheth.

The eagle only has twelve wings, yet each wing has three parts for the three heads. This means each wing represents three religions depending on the head being viewed. (2 Esdras 11:22-23)

One of the wings on the right side rose up to govern the world. After its rule, it vanished completely without a trace. (2 Esdras 11:12) This happened because it attached itself to the power of the government to get its way. The Devil (government) has been there the entire time tempting religious leaders to grab their power. Those who do that fall away from GOD.

Another wing rose up and governed for a long time. It also failed.

The third wing rose up, governed, and then vanished. Each large wing did the same, governing as the earlier ones did before they disappeared. The large wings were the Jews and Christians. (2 Esdras 11:18-19)

Then small wings on the right side began rising up to seize power. Some of them governed briefly and then quickly disappeared. Some wings rose up and were unable to govern at all. The small wings are the alternate religions of Japheth, such as Buddhism, Hinduism, Jainism, etc. (2 Esdras 11:20-21)

After this, some of the small wings left the others and moved under the head on the right side. This signifies the conversion from Middle Eastern religious beliefs while forming Zoroastrianism and Sikhism. These two religions have some form of roots from Muslim-type beliefs and were symbolically under the house of Ham. Zoroastrianism is from Persian origins, and Sikhism has the largest religious military called the Khalsa army. (2 Esdras 11:24)

The four remaining wings were Hinduism, Buddhism, Jainism, and Rastafarianism. These wings plotted to rise up and take power. They used Buddhism first. Buddhism entered the Oriental lands and merged with their religions. They were not successful because they connected with the government while doing so. The next small wing that rose up was Rastafarianism. They didn't last long at all because they claimed that an emperor of one of the nations was Jesus. Their religious foundation was joined to the government, and their reign ended. (2 Esdras 11:25-27)

Jainism and Hinduism remained. While they planned on seizing control, the middle head of the eagle woke up. The middle head is the Jews and the Christians. The middle head joined the other two heads of Ham and Japheth and began taking Jainism and Hinduism down before they could rise. (2 Esdras 11:28-31)

The middle head gained power over the entire world by joining the nations in trickery. The Christians used the nations to gain an oppressive rule over the people. They were leading witch trials, heresy trials, religious wars, and wars for resources and lands. The Christian denominations did this by joining the churches to politics while never getting along with one another. They had Christians in political positions secretly using misinterpretations of the Bible to guide their decisions. (2 Esdras 11:32)

The entire middle head of Shem had destroyed itself by allowing the nations to take complete control. The nations' leaders were in command of the churches while denying GOD, and practiced separation of church and state at the same time.

According to the Bible, Christianity is the Devil's servant. We find the outcome of this behavior in Revelation chapter 12, verse 4. A third of the angels (stars) were cast out of heaven, and one third of the world claimed to be Christian. (Revelation 1:20) They had deceitfully joined the North American government in warring with the Muslims for oil. (2 Esdras 11:33) Christians were cast out of heaven for helping fuel the war.

Ham and Japheth remained. They were both exercising power by being connected to the governments. In this prophecy, Ham then ate Japheth. This is because those who call themselves Muslims war against what they call polytheism. (2 Esdras 11:34-35)

Only Ham remained and was indoctrinated into the Middle Eastern and African governments. The Muslims in those political positions have warred and fought with many people. At this point, Ham's son Canaan is revealed. Canaan is the governments of the nations. They are Cain's house, and together they slew every religion for power. Each religion that attempted to rise up and gain control by holding onto the house of Cain vanished. And though these religions still remain, they have no authority in the governing of heavenly or earthly affairs. The governments have separation of church and state, and they deny GOD. Each religion was used by the nations. The governments made the religions think that they were their friends. After each religion helped the governments succeed over the other religions, the governments denied those who helped them.

As it has been revealed, all of the eagle's rival wings and heads were part of the same body. There were three heads for the three families of Noah and Abraham, and there were twelve wings because each of the three families was split into twelve portions. That is the meaning of the eagle. It fights with itself and destroys its own people. The churches could not see that all religions were part of one body. The eagle was considered a cruel, oppressive ruler because it was merged with the governments. GOD didn't give one religion a blessing and cast the rest out. There are specific blessings that went to each religion. Their blessings came from GOD; what they did with them wasn't.

The Eagle Transforms

The governmental leaders who deny GOD, were also in command of the religions. Because of this, GOD wasn't with the religions, and the eagle aligns to the iron-wielding dragon. The dragon is the Devil and Satan. (2 Esdras 11:36-44)

The entire body of the eagle was found to be worthless because the religions obeyed the Devil. Their entirety and that of the world needs to be renewed. (2 Esdras 11:45-46)

The reason that the heads of the eagle disappeared was because they went under the command of the nations. When they did this, GOD was no longer their head. Once GOD was no longer their head, the nations had no more need for them. Satan (the world political leaders and officers) had taken GOD's authority. They had beheaded GOD's throne. The house of Ham simply disappears with them. (2 Esdras 12:1-25)

The national officials used whatever power the religions offered. When religion seemed to have no more power to offer, the officials discarded them. They used the idea of separation of church and state to push religion off them once they didn't need it anymore.

All these interpretations are simplified and can be far more intricate. More information on the twelve kings spoken of in Second Esdras chapter 12, verses 14-18 can be found in the Seal of the Beast and the Harlot in Chapter 7 of the first book in this series.

The last head of the eagle, which represents the house of Ham, is prophesied to die in its bed. This aligns to the seal of Jezebel. The nations are called Jezebel, and anyone who fornicates with them dies spiritually. Once they are your guide and protector, then GOD isn't your guide and protector anymore. (Revelation 2:18-29) (2 Esdras 12:26-35)

It would have been safer to have just lived on the milk of the Word of GOD. (1 Peter 2:2) (Hebrews 5:13)

At this point, a lion came out of the forest to rebuke the eagle. The lion signifies the Messiah. He rebukes and condemns the nations which are the house of Cain. The nations fused with the religions were the eagle.

The LORD came and sat on HIS throne, which is the direct descendant of the actual Jesus. (Daniel 7:9-14) Those who had gone under the government gave up their birthright and blessing as Edom did. Their birthrights and blessings were sealed to their Akashic Records. Their records were handed over and administered through the LORD's throne.

Previously the eagle spoke from the middle of its body. That means that the people of the religions, as one body, spoke from within their own hearts. (Isaiah 29:13) On December 21st, 2016, the sacred heart of Jesus was connected to the religions so that they could be heard. The eagle then spoke from within the heart of the direct descendant of Jesus. He could feel the LORD inside of his chest as HE communicated. (2 Esdras 11:10)

Step by step, the LORD's Son had to baptize the kingdom in various stages. He baptized the calf, the lion, the bear, the leopard, the dragon, and the eagle.

The eagle must be baptized and reborn. Return to GOD. (Exodus 19:4) (Isaiah 40:31)

The Eagle Transforms

Consider the nations (or empires) throughout history. They eventually collapse. The average lifespan of an empire is said to be 250 years. (Check diverse translations of Tao Te Ching Chapter 57) What they all had in common was that they used military as their leadership. They built their foundations on honor of those who fought their battles. They each solved their problems with weapons. In ancient times they used swords, spears, and bows. Today they use guns and bombs. The Bible teaches us that those who live by the sword will die by the sword. The sword that they live by is used to honor their people of authority. They don't live by that which protects the health of the planet; they live by that which honors and protects their power.

There are thought to be trillions upon trillions of stars in the universe. A great number of those stars have planets orbiting them. Imagine how vast many of those planets are potential life holders. Each life-holding planet is like a nation. Every planet that has a military leadership will collapse. (2 Esdras 14:17)
Though iron is good for you as a vitamin, the iron and the 12-star garland upon the lady's head remind us of a supernova, which is induced through the production of iron in a star. Each nation is also like a star. When the nation becomes a military empire, iron becomes the leader. This means that military-based nations live by the sword. Those who live by the sword also die by the sword. (Revelation 13:10)

Vegans are generally anti-war in disposition. The standard of the vegan mindset is not to kill and therefore doesn't have to live by the sword. Vegans who don't produce iron for war are the light of the nations. They are the light of the world that won't blow up.

When a star produces iron and explodes, the iron remaining from the explosion can be used. Similarly, the lessons we learn and the technology that we gain from the dying nations are still with us.

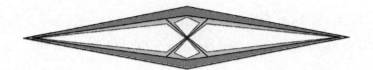

Book of Life Afterward and Epilogue
The Eighth Sinew of Ashes and Manna in Marble and Silver

For thousands of years now, people have wondered how Jesus returns. Some have said that He is coming on the clouds of heaven in the east. That is symbolic, as explained in book 1 of this series.

(Luke 17:20-21) "Now when He was asked by the Pharisees when the kingdom of God would come, He answered them and said, "The kingdom of God does not come with observation; nor will they say, See here!' or 'See there!' For indeed, the kingdom of God is within you.""

This sinew clarifies how Jesus will return. To enter the body of churches, Jesus will present Himself holding the kingdom internally.

To give the churches a chance to listen to GOD, someone must call on the religions. The leaders and followers are to be addressed by a man who has the kingdom within. All twelve houses shall attend. (Matthew 12:25) The speaker is to hold the entire kingdom internally. To assure that the kingdom is inside of Him, He must eat the Livet for at least one year before the presentation.

This conference isn't about the church attendants expressing their religious views. It is their turn to listen with intent. This is about the churches hearing the ideas of the kingdom within. They are all to get along. The information shared is to be about the entire kingdom of GOD as explained within these books.

Each tribe is a different part of the body of people. They each sense in different ways. Each tribe is important.

The Tribe of Levi is the Church of Phillipia and the Legs of the Kingdom.
When He stands near the Tribe of Levi, they will know the kingdom of heaven stands within.

The Tribe of Reuben is the church of Ephesus and the Nose of the Kingdom.
When He comes near the Tribe of Reuben, they will smell the kingdom of heaven within.

187

The Tribe of Dan is the Church of Smyrna and the Fingers of the Kingdom.
When He handles the Tribe of Dan, they will touch the kingdom of heaven within.

The Tribe of Joseph is the Church of Pergamos and the Mouth of the Kingdom.
When He speaks to the Tribe of Joseph, they will recognize the language of the kingdom of heaven within.

The Tribe of Benjamin is the Church of Thyatira and the Arms of the Kingdom.
When He holds the Tribe of Benjamin, they will handle the kingdom of heaven within.

The Tribe of Simeon is the Church of Sardis and the Ears of the Kingdom.
When He speaks to the Tribe of Simeon, they will hear the kingdom of heaven within.

The Tribe of Judah is the Church of Philadelphia and the Mind of the Kingdom.
When He logicizes with the Tribe of Judah, they will comprehend the kingdom of heaven within.

The Tribe of Naphtali is the Church of Laodicea and the Tongue of the Kingdom.
When He feeds the Tribe of Naphtali with the Word of GOD, they will taste the kingdom of heaven within. (John 6:53)

The Tribe of Asher is the Church of Galatia and the Chest of the Kingdom.
When He loves the Tribe of Asher, they will realize the kingdom of heaven within.

The Tribe of Issachar is the Church of Philemo and the Torso of the Kingdom.
When He breathes near the Tribe of Issachar, they will respire the kingdom of heaven within.

The Tribe of Zebulun is the Church of Thessalonia and the Hands of the Kingdom.
When He touches the Tribe of Zebulun, they will feel the kingdom of heaven within.

The Tribe of Gad is the Church of Corinth and the Eyes of the Kingdom.
When He looks at the Tribe of Gad, they will finally see the kingdom of heaven within.

As He speaks with the churches that are gathered together, they will all comprehend as one. This is done with the family of Shem, meaning the Christians and the Jews. Once they comprehend the kingdom within, the family of Japheth will awaken. Japheth is the internal organs of the kingdom. Ham will also awaken.

This is the path of the rebirth of the kingdom of heaven. (John 3:3) That is how to wake them.